REVERSE INFLAMMATION NATURALLY

Michelle Honda PhD

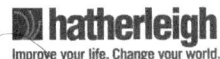

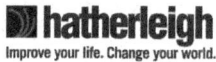
Improve your life. Change your world.

Hatherleigh Press is committed to preserving and protecting the natural resources of the earth. Environmentally responsible and sustainable practices are embraced within the company's mission statement.

Visit us at www.hatherleighpress.com and register online for free offers, discounts, special events, and more.

Reverse Inflammation Naturally
Text Copyright © 2017 Michelle Honda

Library of Congress Cataloging-in-Publication Data is available.
ISBN: 978-1-57826-680-7

All rights reserved. No part of this book may be reproduced, stored in a retrieval system, or transmitted, in any form or by any means, electronic or otherwise, without written permission from the publisher.

DISCLAIMER
Limit of Liability/Disclaimer of Warranty
This book contains nutrition and plant based suggestions. The intention of this book is to complement a person's current treatment plan. The author recognizes a qualified physician or health care professional should be consulted regarding your specific complaint. The author does not recommend self-diagnosis or treatment. The publisher and author specifically disclaim any and all liability occurring directly or indirectly from the application of any information contained in this book.

Printed in the United States

Follow Michelle Honda PhD on Facebook:
www.facebook.com/NewHopeForCrohnsAndColitis

To learn lots about nutrition and healthy living, and for more information on her private practice, visit Michelle's blog:
www.michellehonda.com

DEDICATION

To all the people embarking on a path to phenomenal health.

ACKNOWLEDGEMENTS

To BEGIN WITH, I would like to acknowledge my patients who embraced a new dietary approach to healing. I applaud their willingness to adopt the necessary lifestyle changes and to further understand the importance of preventive care and the role of complementary medicine. Their desire to heal and regain independence inspires me to continue to deepen my knowledge to be of better service.

First, and foremost, I wish to thank the exceptionally skilled and talented team from Hatherleigh Press. I among other authors and readers who are indebted to this team for providing invaluable resources, making it possible for people to learn about preventive health maintenance and the science of complementary medicine.

I especially wish to thank my publisher Andrew Flach for his superb expertise and guidance. I have deep appreciation to the entire Hatherleigh team, in particular Ryan Kennedy, Ryan Tumambing, and Anna Krusinski for their wonderful support and knowledge.

I am deeply grateful and appreciative to Dr. Ellen Tart-Jensen whose unflagging support is never irresolute. You can read more about Ellen Tart-Jensen Ph.D. at www.bernardjensen.com.

Without the work of other researchers and scientists, I would not have the broad base of knowledge to draw from and further extend it to my patients. Along with these specialists and other physicians, they have availed to us natural medicine and human cell biology to better understand the disease and healing process.

And lastly but not least, my husband, Ron, who is always supportive and patient, as we continue on in this life's journey.

CONTENTS

Foreword by Ellen Tart-Jensen, Ph.D., D.Sc.   xi
Preface   xv
Introduction   xvii

CHAPTER 1
An Overview of Inflammation   1

Stages of Inflammation
  Acute Inflammation
  Chronic Inflammation
  Conventional Treatment for Chronic Inflammation
  Symptoms of Inflammation

Inflammation Pathways
  Role of Prostaglandins (PG) and Linoleic Fats verses Dietary Fats
  Essential Fatty Acids and Inflammation
  Delta-6-Desaturase
  Case Study: Reversing Eczema

The Immune System: Key Player in the Inflammation Process
  Medications Compete with the Immune System
  Effect of Steroid Drugs on the Immune System
  Neu5Gc and Arachidonic Acid

Food and Plant Properties Create Immune Imbalance
  Nightshade Vegetables and Fruits Cause Inflammation
  Nightshades Can Be Toxic
  How to Test for Sensitivity
  Chili Peppers

Case Histories: Food Related Autoimmune Disorders and Inflammation
  Common Triggers
  Full Manifestation of Rheumatoid Arthritis Involving Nicotine

v

Thyroiditis and Gluten
Fibromyalgia
   Fibromyalgia and Gluten
   Fibrin and Proteolytic Enzymes
   Hypertension May Coincide with Circulating Fibrin

CHAPTER 2
Illnesses Related to Inflammation   15
Heart Disease
   What Food is Causing Inflammation in the Arteries?
Cancer
   Angiogenesis
Diabetes
   Obesity
   Insulin Resistance and Inflammation
   Leptin Hormone
Autism
   Treating Autism with Flavonoids
Metabolic Syndrome
   Effects of Diet on Metabolic Syndrome
Asthma, Allergy and Sinusitis
   Reducing Mucus through Diet
   Boosting the Immune System

CHAPTER 3
Key Players of the Inflammatory Response   27
Omega-3 EFAs
   The Problem with Omega-6 EFAs
Oil Production Process
   Grapeseed Oil Process
   Rapeseed (Canola) Oil

Olive Oil
Coconut Oil
Free Radicals Affect Disease and Inflammation
Free Radicals and Antioxidants
Candida Causes Inflammation
Recommendations for Combating Candida

CHAPTER 4
Foods and Substances that Trigger Inflammation   35
Foods to Avoid
Artificial Sweeteners
Irradiated Food
Nitrate and Nitrites
Trans Fats
Acrylamide
Free Radicals from Pesticides
Environmental Chemicals

CHAPTER 5
Foods That Reduce Inflammation   43
Teas to Help Reduce Inflammation
Matcha Tea
Tulsi Tea
Sage Tea
Kombucha Tea

CHAPTER 6
Assess Your Personal Health Status   49
Does Your Body Need to Be Propped Up?
Examples of Conditions Related to a Nutrient Deficiency
Assess Your Level of Nutrition

CHAPTER 7
Natural Supplementation for Reversing Inflammation 55
Minerals
Vitamins
   Vitamin C
   Vitamin A
   Vitamin D (Fat Soluble)
   Vitamin D (Water Soluble)
   Vitamin E
   Vitamin K2 (MK-7)
Essential Fatty Acids (EFAs)
Gut Flora
Antioxidants
   Alpha Lipoic Acid
   Beta-Carotene (and Other Carotenoids)
   Astaxanthin
   Falcarinol
   Lycopene
   Resveratrol
   Sulphur Phyto-Nutrients
   Bromelain
   Epigallocatechin-3-gallate (EGCG)
   A-Adenosyl Methionine (SAMe)
Proteolytic Enzymes
   Serrapeptase and Proteinase
   Nattokinase Enzyme
   Superoxide Dismutase (SOD) Enzyme

CHAPTER 8
Purchasing Herbal and Supplement Products   67

Choosing a Quality Herbal Product
How to Choose a Quality Supplement
Look for Tested Formulas
Look for Quality Ingredients
Look for Chemical Additives
Look for Source Absorbability Factor
How to Make Tea Using Plant Parts

CHAPTER 9
Reversing Inflammation—Naturally   73

Anti-Inflammatory Herbs
Shosaikoto
Curcumin
Boswellia
Cat's Claw
Horseweed (Conyza Canadensis)
Devil's Claw (Harpagophytum procumbens)
Sinomenine (Sinomenium acutum)
White Willow Bark
Shiitake Mushrooms
Cayenne Pepper (Capsaicin)
Rhein (Rhubarb)
Skullcap (Scutellaria baicalensis)
Glycyrrhizin (Licorice Root Extract)
Ginger
Garlic

CHAPTER 10
Diet Therapy for Reversing Inflammation 83

Smoothies

    Popular Smoothie Ingredients

Juicing

    Partner Your Ingredients to Suit Your Digestion

    Popular Juice Ingredients

    Juice Preparation

    Green Juices

    Wheat Grass

    Adding Protein to Liquids

    Dietary Fiber

Pro-Inflammatory Sweeteners

    Natural Fruit Sugar

    Additional Healthy Sweeteners

Daily Meal Plan for Reversing Inflammation

    General Rules

    A Few Personal Diet Recommendations

    Daily Menu Plan

CHAPTER 11
Recipes 97

    Anti-Inflammatory Cocktails

    Fruit Juice Recipes

    Blended Drinks and Smoothie Recipes

    Soups and Salads

    Dinner

Conclusion 113

Resources 114

Bibliography 116

About the Author 121

FOREWORD

From time to time, there will appear in the arena of natural healing a unique individual who makes a tremendous contribution to his or her field. Dr. Michelle Honda is just such an individual. I have had the opportunity to know Dr. Honda personally for many years as a student, professional colleague, and friend. Having healed herself through nutritional measures from her own inflammatory conditions, Dr. Honda began a long journey of formal educational studies including nutrition and natural medicine, earning her Ph.D. in order to serve and teach others to get well. She has now worked in private practice with thousands of patients, observing what works and what doesn't work to help people regain their health. Dr. Honda is one of the most sincere, concerned doctors I know of in our times. Not only does she make a huge difference in the lives of her patients, she is also contributing tremendously by sharing her depth of knowledge and experience by writing several life-saving books. Now she has written another treasure, *Reverse Inflammation Naturally*.

In our busy world filled with all the modern conveniences—computers, telephones, cell phones, tablets, televisions, cars, planes, boats, and trains—people are more exhausted than they have ever been. Pollution is at an all-time high. People are frantic and hurried. Practically gone are the times for the family meal with foods brought in from the garden and prepared wholesomely. In order to keep up with the fast-paced world, people are eating fast foods filled with preservatives, starches, grease, sugars, and chemicals. They feel tired so they live on highly caffeinated beverages during the day and alcohol to relax at night. Almost ninety percent of our population is taking some form of medication. The result is *inflammation*.

Inflammation is at the root of all illnesses that plague humankind today. Inflammation comes as a result of extreme daily stress, adrenal fatigue, elevated glucose levels, heavy metals and chemicals in the body, and many other conditions that Dr. Honda explains in an easy to understand manner throughout this wonderful book. If you have pain or swelling in the tissues, muscles, or joints; suffer from acid reflux; or have any form of cardiovascular disease, blood clots, high blood pressure, elevated cholesterol levels, auto-immune disease, diabetes, cancer, ADHD, autism, migraines, digestive issues, thyroiditis, sinus infections, eczema, allergies, or asthma this book is for you. The recommendations in this book are what you have long been waiting for.

This book is a step-by-step guide to teach you how to move out of the painful condition into having energy and feeling well again. Dr. Bernard Jensen, whom I studied with and Dr. Honda learned from as well, used to say, "We need to put new tissue in place of old and we do that by the way we eat, drink, think, and live." If you have been living a fast-paced life filled with stress and eating foods that are not pure, whole, and natural you have built your disease. No amount of medication is going to be able to unravel or "cure" your condition. As a matter of fact, anti-inflammatory drugs only relieve the symptom for a short time and then cause huge side effects in the long run. Many of you are experiencing those side effects now.

In this book, Dr. Honda will explain to you the difference between acute and chronic, long-term inflammation. She will tell you what causes both, as well as teach you about the illnesses that occur as a result. She will show you how the immune system is a key player in the inflammation process and explain how medications are composed of toxic chemicals that disrupt the immune system and become very difficult for the body to eliminate. Many people as I write this are suffering from what they think is a mysterious illness such as fibromyalgia or rheumatoid arthritis, to name just a few. Doctors have told them they have medicine to help them ease the pain, but that it cannot be cured. They are taking the medicines because they don't know what else to do, but the medicines are causing problems such as difficulty sleeping, constipation, headaches, or any myriad of side effects. People are losing hope.

Reverse Inflammation Naturally is a book about hope. It will not only show you the causes of your ailments, it will supply you with the inflammatory foods you should avoid and teach you about the foods that reduce inflammation and help to heal the body. If you have hypertension, it will provide some amazing botanicals that lower blood pressure and relax the vessels to free them from inflammation. If you have high cholesterol, it will teach you which fats to avoid as well as healthy fats to consume. If you are fatigued, it will help you improve your thyroid, adrenal, and nerve function so you may have energy again. It will give you specific herbal remedies, vitamins, and minerals that have proven through research to be powerful anti-inflammatories without side effects. Finally, you will be able to take your health and your life into your own hands. You might find that something you have been doing for years like consuming artificial sweeteners or nightshade vegetables, coupled with stress, caused your illness. Now you can let all of the things go that created the pain and know which foods and drinks to consume to build new healthy tissue in your body. Delicious recipes and meal plans are provided to make the journey easier.

This book is truly a gift for all who are searching for health. It is also a wonderful manual for doctors, nurses, nutritionists, naturopaths, acupuncturists, or chiropractors who wish to have the best up-to-date research and information on ways to help their patients reverse the inflammatory response. For the one seeking health, it will be like a visit to Dr. Honda herself as she guides you and explains to you what to do on a daily basis to feel better.

—Ellen Tart-Jensen, Ph.D., D.Sc., CCII, author of *Health is Your Birthright: How to Create the Health You Deserve*

PREFACE

It is not uncommon for people to shrug off their day-to-day aches and pains, or to ignore the fact that they knowingly eat items that are unhealthy. The public at large is still in the dark when it comes to the repercussions of food and other substances routinely eaten, as well as what may be manifesting throughout their body.

A common area where many people *do* have some sense of concern is their medication intake. Even though commercials convey the problems of drug side effects, they do not offer any other options, so people are at a loss for what else to do to minimize their discomfort.

And for most people, the ways in which inflammation spreads and develops is clouded with mystery. It is this lack of knowledge and understanding of inflammation and its role in the disease process that has led me to write this book. In these pages, we will seek to explain not only the pathways and processes that inflammation takes, but the myriad of ways in which we enhance and reinforce inflammation in our daily lives. We will also learn how to quell and reverse the spread of inflammation in the body by addressing the causes and making simple diet adjustments.

There are many facets to inflammation. This book will discuss the different stages and specific types of inflammation associated with certain disease conditions and complaints, which, in turn, will reveal much about its progression in the body. It is my hope that, by doing so, it will allow you to peer into your body on a cellular level, where you can observe how your inflammatory/immune system silently harms and disrupts your optimum state of health. Equally as important is an understanding of how certain drugs negatively affect the anti-inflammatory pathways and how they stop the liver's ability to appropriately clean itself.

The public at large is most interested in the causes of their conditions and what can be done to ease their pain. Yet traditional medicine often fails to provide this information. You yourself may be reading this book because you are seeking answers. The catalysts for disease and illness presented in this book are drawn from my own practice and experience in healing my patients. The causes presented are the ones most often to blame, and the recommendations and solutions offered are those that have shown to be the most effective.

Armed with the knowledge that one must treat the body as a whole if one is to achieve lasting health and wellness, the solutions presented throughout this book are those that treat inflammation with natural medicine. Remain mindful of the fact that our health is integrally linked to the world around us. Let us not forget that these herbs and extracts have been used for food and medicine for as long as humans have occupied this earth. The use of plants as medicine and food has been passed down through the ages for our *benefit*, not our detriment. Natural based medicine is perfect for those individuals who have suffered at the hands of medication side effects in the past, or who have avoided seeking treatment for their ailments due to fear of the same. And for anyone wishing to lower their medication dosage (or eliminate the need for it altogether), natural medicine provides a safe alternative, especially when there have been consistent complications in one's current medication treatment plan.

In addition, I've provided a number of diet and food suggestions for day-to-day eating that can more quickly reduce your inflammation. To help you get started, there are also recommended meal plans and juice and meal recipes.

In reading this book, I wish to impress upon you your own ability to live a happy, healthy life. My goal is to remove frustration by providing an understanding of the disease process—and the process for positive change that can be built on as you progress towards a happy and healthy future.

—Michelle Honda Ph.D., D.Sc.

INTRODUCTION

Americans are in the midst of a health crisis, one that may rival even those in third world countries. Yet society as a whole seems to have adopted a cavalier attitude toward prescribed medications and food consumption habits, to the detriment of their short- and long-term health.

America is now being hailed as the "Inflammation Nation." As a result of regularly ingesting non-steroidal anti-inflammatory drugs (NSAIDs), such as Advil, Aleve, Bayer, Motrin, Excedrin and ibuprofen, many people have become at risk of developing stomach problems involving nausea and pain due to inflammation. The continued usage of these over-the-counter painkillers creates inflammation throughout the stomach and the intestines, which in turn escalates the need for an alternative to pain medication. These conditions often escalate to the more serious complaints of ulcers, gut disorders, acid reflux and increased levels of *H. pylori*.

A study performed in 2010 by the American Gastroenterological Association discovered that over 30 million Americans took over-the-counter medication (NSAIDs) on a daily basis for the relief of pain.[1] Add several cups of coffee to this routine, and you have a fast track to gastric ulcers.

We can no longer afford to hide from the chronic illnesses that our dreadful eating habits have created and exacerbated. Inflammation, initiated by unhealthy lifestyle choices, is believed to be a main driving force for the development of the deadliest cancers, heart diseases, skin diseases, dementia, arthritic conditions, and many more.

But inflammation is not necessarily the core concern.

In order for any disease to manifest, there must first be a set of circumstances in place that sets the stage. At some point, the body must have become imbalanced through a series of events that produced malfunctioning systems, toxicity, and fatigue. In some (though not all) instances, the body will let you know through physical indicators that inflammation is taking hold. But relying on your body to tell you when a problem has already started is an imperfect method of detection and disease prevention.

---

1 American Gastroenterological Association. "Patient Center: NSAIDS." April 2010.

Staying healthy has been an obsession of mine ever since I first introduced vegetable juice into my dietary routine, back in my twenties. I soon recognized that I had made a choice, one which would support my living longer, avoiding chronic illnesses, and remaining active well into my advanced years.

That same choice, and others like it, is open to everyone.

Professionally, I strive to be of assistance to others by sharing the many exciting advancements in disease prevention and safe, alternative approaches in treatment care. This book, like others I have written, embodies my commitment to helping others learn about these new discoveries while empowering them with all the tools necessary to bring themselves back to a state of vibrant health.

The Holistic Approach to Reversing Inflammation

I, like many other doctors, scientists, and health practitioners, am all too aware of the ills associated with inflammation. Depending on the healing modality, the treatment approaches for inflammation are as varied and widespread as are the cultures around the world.

In my practice, I work from a holistic approach, and in doing so have observed hundreds of chronic inflammation cases. In these cases, my treatment protocol always centers on removing the individual or interconnected causes of the complaint. By taking away the primary instigators, our own immune systems are allowed a much-needed break, which serves as an effective foundation for future treatment methods.

We then assess the patient's medication regimen and their possible long- or short-term side effects. This area must be addressed for a few reasons.

In the industrialized world that we live in, the majority of the public have become accustomed to taking over-the-counter or prescription medications for all of their health complaints. This in and of itself poses a health risk, especially in cases of inflammation, since the inflammation pathways are also used to detoxify and repair the body. On a daily basis, this system eliminates toxins in the air we breathe, removes metabolic waste and built-up toxins in our tissues, and repairs cells that have been injured. But these crucial pathways are suppressed by medication, as well as those responsible for cellular detoxification.

Another common side effect is liver damage, brought on by the liver's inability to detoxify appropriately, resulting in liver toxicity. (This is why anyone placed on a prescription anti-inflammatory medication is also issued cyclic liver blood tests to ensure proper liver function.) To effectively treat patients and quicken the healing process—without causing liver damage—holistic medicine employs natural whole substances derived from plants and nature to replace any current or future need for pain medication in a patient.

Finally, we investigate the patient's current health status, which may include a variety of immune triggers and internal weaknesses or imbalances. Areas commonly discussed include:

- All symptom complaints and current disease conditions
- Diet (foods and liquids routinely consumed)
- Known foods or substances that cause discomfort
- Lifestyle habits (good and bad)
- Any healthy supplementation external to diet
- Stress levels and coping ability
- Exercise
- Occupation
- Medications
- Main challenges
- Ultimate goal

Also considered when putting together a case history is their level of happiness, their life goals, and their hopes for their future, whether related to career, health, or the ability to be healthy and enjoy retirement life. While listening to a person explain why they have come to see me and in learning about their lifestyle as a whole, a list is quickly formulated about what this person requires in the way of nutrient support and diet adjustments. Depending on specific symptom complaints, patients also learn about contributing factors involved in the manifestation of their problem, along with natural, alternative solutions that are safe and effective in alleviating their current pain and suffering—all without the assistance of drugs.

> **Cause and Confusion**
>
> Not every professional agrees with the current understanding of the causes of and remedies for inflammation (despite the massive amounts of literature substantiating these claims). In some cases, this is an issue of interpretation—an issue of claims being too definitive or too general. Regardless, this confusion over cause and effect has prompted some scientists to state that foods commonly associated with certain conditions have *no* anti-inflammatory benefit or cause, and that inflammation is simply related to the processes of disease pathology and bad health habits. They insist that the only reason for reduced inflammation after ingesting certain foods or natural compounds is not the chemicals found in plants, but is rather a result of a reduction of animal protein and lower calorie content.
>
> There are more studies taking place today on plant chemistry than ever before. But when compared to the amount of research studies performed in pharmacology for the production of drugs, the number of studies showing the benefit of whole natural substances (which, of course, cannot be patented) is exponentially fewer.
>
> In my personal and professional experience, the claim that certain foods (and properties therein) will not have a positive effect on the body has emphatically not been the case. Regardless of any technical reasons that may cast these results in doubt, I have witnessed the myriad ways that specific foods, and the properties in food and plants, can have a profound effect on the symptoms of disease complaints. There *is* worth in learning to recognize the triggers for inflammation and disease conditions that may be found in food and plants, but learning to take advantage of the *curative* powers in the whole, unadulterated substances found in nature is just as impactful in reversing negative health complaints.

The Goal of this Book

The focus of this book, as the title suggests, is to learn how to reverse the inflammation that results from many disease complaints in a wholesome and natural way. The causes and symptom triggers mentioned throughout this book are the same as those I deal with most and have had the greatest success in treating and reversing.

Many times when the cause is dealt with, the majority of the battle is over. This is the main difference between holistic and allopathic treatment protocols. That said, it is important to bear in mind that systems become dysfunctional for many reasons. When a patient has a complaint, it is important to remember that it is *not* all in your head. When we experience chronic stress, for example, the cortisol levels in the body drop, which allows for enhanced inflammation and leaves us more vulnerable to colds and flu.

Realize that physical illnesses, especially those that cannot be easily explained, are the result of multifaceted, neuroendocrine responses. In spite of the manner in which symptoms have manifested in the body, they are created by the mind, brain and body—*together*.

And that is where the holistic approach really shines. Because things *aren't* always that simple; to achieve optimum results, the person and body must be treated as a whole. Regardless of what you may or may not know about physiology, our internal environment is a constant working miracle that is never separate from itself.

In this book, you will learn how to restore a tired, weak body and an overworked immune system. As you make your way through this book, you may start to visualize how something that is taken into the stomach can end up manifesting as pain in an entirely different area of the body (such as an enzyme, called solanine, which causes rheumatoid arthritis).

The information presented here is drawn from a number of sources, including the latest discoveries regarding anti-inflammatory properties found in foods, spices and herbs around the globe. My goal for this book is to assist you in fully restoring your health and provide for any direction your future may take you. By applying my recommendations, you will find yourself on the road to optimal health.

CHAPTER 1

An Overview of Inflammation

INFLAMMATION HAS RAPIDLY gained a bad reputation, but you may be surprised to learn that inflammation is among your body's best friends. Inflammation works to stave off the constant bombardment of unwanted pathogens that are part of our everyday environment. Created via the cells and substances in our immune system, inflammation allows the body to ward off and defeat potentially harmful viruses, bacteria, and fungi.

Inflammation operates much like the smoke alarms in our homes. Whenever we injure ourselves or cause a break or damage to our outer protective layer (the skin), our immune system sets in motion a series of defense mechanisms to clot the blood (to stop bleeding) and inflame the surrounding tissue (to destroy any bacteria that has seeped into the wound).

Stages of Inflammation

Acute Inflammation
In the early stages of immune response, the body sends out an alarm signal, which produces a series of symptoms. Described as acute, these symptoms are characterized by heat, impaired function, pain, reddening of tissue, and swelling.

Even though the acute stage of inflammation may affect performance of certain duties, its symptoms and effects are only temporary. Tissue normally heals anywhere within a few minutes to a few days; depending on the injury, mobility returns fairly quickly. An example of an acute inflammation response is what you would expect to see from a small cut or scrape.

Chronic Inflammation
Chronic inflammation, on the other hand, signifies something entirely different. When the body has been struggling for a long time, unable to effectively protect itself, chronic inflammation can take hold, as the body continues to fight a losing battle against infection or imbalance.

Unlike the acute form of inflammation, as chronic inflammation takes hold in our bodies, a sequence of cellular changes takes place. During this time, our inflammatory processes actually work against our body, often leading to tissue damage. The science behind these interactions is somewhat complex, but in simple terms, the cells involved with inflammation and our immune response are white blood cells (lymphocytes, neutrophils) and macrophages. Other, complementary systems participating in the inflammatory response consist of prostaglandins (PGE2-PGI2), histamine, leukotrienes, serotonin and bradykinin.

Chronic inflammation has been shown to be the main factor in heart disease, obesity, type 2 diabetes, dementia, Alzheimer's, chronic fatigue, autoimmune diseases, rheumatoid arthritis, fibromyalgia and chronic bronchitis—to name but a few of the serious complications that can arise from uncontrolled inflammation.

Conventional Treatment for Chronic Inflammation
Conventional medicine is aware of the many driving forces behind chronic inflammation, but is not employing any treatment strategies other than prescription medications that overwhelm the body's systems. As Dr. Zoltan Rona points out, "While short use of steroidal and non-steroidal anti-inflammatory drugs can be very effective, long-term use of any of these drugs (beyond a few weeks) can lead to life-threatening side effects (hemorrhage, osteoporosis, heart disease)."[2]

Symptoms of Inflammation
Most people are fully aware of what their degree of pain is at any given time, and are usually aware of any degenerative diseases they may be currently dealing with. Examples may include certain forms of arthritis, chronic skin disorders (psoriasis, scleroderma), lupus, thyroiditis, or any other complaint that involves a chronic form of inflammation.

But what if there *are* no noticeable signs? The following lab tests can assist in determining if it is time to start implementing lifestyle changes:

---

[2] Zoltan P. Rona, Reversing Chronic Inflammation: Vitality Magazine, November 2012.

- Elevated levels of erythrocyte sedimentation rate (ESR)
- High sensitivity C-reactive protein (hs-CRP)
- White blood cell levels
- Fibrin and rouleau formation (red blood cells stacking on each other)

Inflammation Pathways

Role of Prostaglandins (PG) and Linoleic Fats vs. Dietary Fats
Inflammation is regulated by a group of diverse, hormone-like active lipid compounds called prostaglandins (PGE2[3] and PGI2). Prostaglandins are derived from fatty acids that are produced in many locations throughout the body (whereas endocrine hormones are produced at a specific site in the human body). Both inflammation and endocrine pathways can be stimulated or depressed, depending on signals produced in the body.

Essential Fatty Acids and Inflammation
Essential fatty acids have an enormous effect on pro-inflammatory prostaglandins. Our diet has a profound effect on inflammation since the body makes prostaglandins from fatty acids. For this reason, providing your body with extra supplementation of specific fats will bring about tremendous relief for certain health conditions like chronic eczema; however, most people's dietary fat and oil intake is a key contributor when it comes to prolonged inflammation and diseases like cancer. For example, vegetable oils should be excluded from your diet as much as possible; that, and the elimination of all sources of trans-fatty acids and foods that may contain them, like chips and processed food, is a great first step to getting your inflammation under control. These types of fats stimulate inflammatory prostaglandins. (Sources include margarine, partially hydrogenated vegetable oils, and vegetable shortening.)

To produce inhibitory prostaglandins, try to enrich your diet with gamma linolenic acids (GLAs) and other omega 3 fatty acids. Excellent choices include evening primrose oil, currant oil, flax seed oil and borage oil. Those omega 3 fatty acids that are especially beneficial can be found in anchovies, sardines, herring, Alaskan salmon, and oily fish (such as mack-

---

[3] Prostaglandin E2 (PGE2) is a principal link between inflammation and degenerative and chronic diseases.

erel). Supplementation of these fats is necessary for counteracting all forms of inflammation and for proper body functioning.

Delta-6-Desaturase

Delta-6-desaturase is an enzyme that plays a critical role in the conversion of chemicals that control a variety of body functions, but it is oftentimes seen as impaired in the chemistries of some individuals. This enzyme works hand in hand with prostaglandins.(Prostaglandins belong to the bioflavonoid family, where they are used for nerve transmission, the immune system and platelet response, and much more.)

Delta-6-desaturase is key to the proper performance of many processes throughout the body. A few examples include maintaining blood pressure and cholesterol levels, digestion, sex hormone synthesis, fluid retention, and blood levels of omega-6 essential fatty acids. Factors that can inhibit D6D include elements in one's environment or certain conditions within the body, such as diabetes, alcohol dependency, and radiation.

Because the enzyme D6D is so uniquely tied into the inadequate production of anti-inflammatory prostaglandins (and severe cases of eczema), I will describe how this interrelationship works. Eczema is often associated with D6D weakness. Treatment for severe cases of eczema almost always involves the support of this weak enzyme. The pro-inflammatory prostaglandin pathways continue to work, which results in a chronic imbalance in these hormone-like compounds, producing heightened inflammation. Basically, the fat storage cells of the body are thrown out of balance and require supplemental support to right themselves.

To reverse this condition (or to serve as a preventive measure), I usually recommend the application of the essential fatty acid found in evening primrose oil, which serves to prop up the impaired enzyme. Known as gamma linolenic acid (GLA), this supportive ingredient allows the body to bypass these blocked enzymes. Specific nutrients and body processes are important in regulating D6D and overseeing the conversion of GLA to prostaglandins, including ascorbic acid, pyridoxine, zinc, vitamin B3, and the pineal hormone melatonin.

I suggest taking 1200 mg of evening primrose oil three times a day if the condition is very troublesome. In the initial stages of treatment, prick open capsules and put directly onto any affected and surrounding areas. This way, the beneficial linoleic acids are more quickly absorbed.

Case Study: Reversing Eczema
As mentioned, evening primrose oil is wonderful for resolving eczema problems (borage works, as well). The reason for this is because the GLAs found in evening primrose oil bypasses certain weak enzymes and directly supports the natural anti-inflammatory prostaglandins.

Other causes of eczema—those related to allergies, dairy, and gluten—may require additional healing approaches. Start with eliminating dairy, and work through any others potential triggers like gluten, citrus, eggs, chocolate, aspartame, and wheat until you find what's exacerbating your condition. To assist in this, have an allergy test performed to help determine your particular intolerances. Finally, make sure to follow the other guidelines expressed in this book for reducing inflammation; in particular, any anti-inflammatory diet recommendations.

For a more rounded program, consider the following recommendations:
- Supplement with raw juices, including carrots, greens and beets
- Antioxidants are extremely beneficial, as is vitamin A for healing and reducing inflammation
- Quercetin (500 mg three times day), probiotics (daily), zinc (25 mg), magnesium (150 mg three times a day), vitamin D (1000 IU twice a day), B complex (100 mg), liquid iodine (2 drops three times a day), fish oil (1000 mg twice a day) and herbs such as Astragalus, fresh cilantro tea, and burdock root can all provide some benefit
- Depending on severity, glutathione and colostrum can offer extra immune support in the short term
- As stress is a normal companion to any hot itchy skin condition, drinking calming teas or taking tinctures to relax all reactive systems can be beneficial. Examples include skullcap, passionflower, St. John's wort, valerian and chamomile.

The Immune System: Key Player in the Inflammation Process

The important thing to understand when dealing with our immune system is that it is affected by nearly everything we do. Even the simple act of overeating suppresses our protective system while promoting an inflammatory response. In learning to control and reverse inflammation naturally, we must first learn how to help our bodies *without* disabling this system.

Medications Compete with the Immune System
Too often, the first step taken to suppress inflammation is through the application of anti-inflammatory drugs. However, these substances not only obstruct the immune system itself, they are also composed of toxic chemicals, which the body must then work to eliminate. These medications are then removed from the body through the same pathways used for primary inflammation. Since detoxification follow the same pathways as inflammation, and these pathways are being obstructed *by* the medication to be eliminated, you end up with an immune system roadblock.

Effect of Steroid Drugs on the Immune System
The ideal immune system is one that works well and is in balance with the rest of the body. But what happens when chemical substances are taken to create an artificial state of balance, such as when certain medications are prescribed to treat autoimmune disorders?

Prednisone and other steroid-type medications are commonly given to patients with an autoimmune disease. Their purpose is to shut off your immune system, which creates a significant imbalance in the way the system works.

In order to understand this imbalance, let's take a brief look at how the immune system works at a granular level.

The immune system operates both from within and outside the cell through the use of a pair of "helper cells." Th-1, or T helper-1, cells work from inside the cell, protecting and warding off pathogens such as bacteria, viruses and mycoplasms (immobile microorganisms thought to be a primitive form of bacteria), while Th-2 (T helper-2) cells guard against invaders from outside the cell wall.

When healthy, this system remains balanced. But when one side or the other becomes weaker or stronger, a serious problem can develop. This is because the Th-1 cells help *control* Th-2 activity; when imbalanced, as is the case with steroidal medications, the Th-1 cells become weaker while the Th-2 cells become overactive. Steroidal medications promote Th-2 cell over-activation, as external threats are seen as more pressing when treating autoimmune disorders. In addition, exposure to toxins from our environment and conditions such as leaky gut syndrome, infections, mercury from flu shots and vaccines, mycoplasma (bacteria), poor digestion, and other medications will also enhance Th-2 cell over-activation.

Neu5Gc and Arachidonic Acid
The monosaccharide Neu5Gc has come under scrutiny as a potential culprit for causing inflammation. While humans no longer manufacture Neu5Gc in their bodies naturally, we do still produce a closely related version called Neu5Ac. That said, we still acquire substantial amounts of Neu5Gc through ingesting red meat from animals that *do* still produce the compound. When the Neu5Gc antibodies that many people have circulating in their blood interacts with Neu5Ac, it sets the stage for chronic inflammation that could easily lead to cancer (there are certain tissues in our body that react to Neu5Gc in ways that lead to accelerated growth).

Studies have been conducted to determine whether red meat or eggs should be removed from the diet to reduce inflammation. In particular, these studies have examined the role that Arachidonic acid plays in our system. Arachidonic acid is an essential omega-6 fatty acid that works with both omega-3 and omega-6 fatty acids. When there are sufficient levels of omega-3's circulating in the blood, arachidonic acid levels are lowered in our tissues. At first glance, one would think this element would cause a problem, since it follows the inflammatory pathways in the body.

To really understand the inflammatory process as it relates to arachidonic acid, a close look at the inflammation pathways and the multiple roles arachidonic acid performs in the body is needed. It is important to realize that, although arachidonic acid is classified as a pro-inflammatory substance, it is equally important in its role as an anti-inflammatory. In studies, even when there were high levels of arachidonic acid coupled with higher levels of long-chain omega-3 fatty acids, inflammation markers were still lower.[4] In fact, epidemiological studies do not show the diet to have any noticeable effect for increasing the production of inflammatory substances in the body.

Food and Plant Properties Create Immune Imbalance

Nightshade Vegetables and Fruits Cause Inflammation
Auto-immune disorders such as rheumatoid arthritis and fibromyalgia, as well as general pain and swelling of the joints, are often an end product

---
4 Luigi Ferrucci, Relationship of Plasma Polyunsaturated Fatty Acids to Circulating Inflammatory Markers. J Clin. Endocrinol Metab, 2006 Feb: 91(2): 439-46, Epub 2005, Oct.18.

of certain properties found in one's diet. In this section, to demonstrate the effects of elimination diets, we'll be taking rheumatoid arthritis as our test case.

Rheumatoid arthritis is classified as an autoimmune disease, an ailment in which the body attacks its own tissue. A primary trigger of most rheumatoid arthritis complaints has shown to be a delayed food allergy, itself a problem related to abnormal gut permeability. As the frequency of intolerances build, inflammation increases throughout the intestinal lining. In much the same way as other gut dysbiosis conditions, unwanted substances seeps through the intestinal wall into the blood and triggers an immune response.[5]

When looking to treat rheumatoid arthritis through one's diet, pay special attention to the items you are eating most often, along with the location of the inflammation, swelling and stiffness, or any abdominal discomfort. Isolated areas are often a clue to the type of problem that may be manifesting.

Nightshades Can Be Toxic

Nightshade (botanical name: Solanaceae) is a family of flowering plants whose properties can have a profoundly negative effect on the body. For example, nicotine (and nicotine compounds like solanine and solanadine) is a property found in nightshade plants, vegetables, and fruits (such as berries) that can become toxic when consumed in large quantities by individuals who are sensitive. These toxins overwhelm the body and attack the nervous system. Signs of physical distress include intestinal pain, arthritic symptoms, diarrhea, vomiting, abdominal pain, headaches and dizziness. Solanine, an alkaloid toxin, is also associated with neurological problems and intestinal disorders.

Common members of the nightshade family include tomato, potato, eggplant, peppers (bell pepper), chili peppers (as well as paprika), goji berry, gooseberry, blueberries and tobacco.

If you find your digestive/nervous system to be very sensitive to this plant species, extend your list to exclude all nightshade as a precautionary treatment plan. Some people only notice a slight amount of discomfort in

---

5 Be aware that people suffering with rheumatoid arthritis may have lower blood levels of folic acid, zinc and protein. Another area to look into is the side effects of medications, which may be causing biochemical changes that have created a need for specific nutrients.

their joints (such as stiffness), while others experience progressive and more intense symptoms, indicating their immune system is functioning poorly.

How to Test for Sensitivity
The most direct way to determine whether you may be sensitive to the nightshade family is to remove all nightshades from your diet. If you do not get a reaction within 48 hours, remain on this version of your elimination diet for several weeks. If these foods were the culprits perpetuating your discomfort, there will be noticeable improvement.

When reintroducing nightshades back into your diet, eat them with each meal (breakfast, lunch and dinner) for 48 hours. If you start to experience pain and discomfort, consider permanently discontinuing these food items.

Chili Peppers
In transitioning away from nightshades, it can be difficult to replace the flavors of certain foods like tomatoes and peppers. Thankfully, the flavor and heat that chili peppers offer is not quite as hard to duplicate. For heat and flavor, add black peppercorns (cracked or ground), wasabi (a Japanese horseradish blend), freshly-ground ginger, or garlic (garlic freshly pressed through a garlic press is hot as well as pungent) to your diet.

Case Histories: Food Related Autoimmune Disorders and Inflammation

The following are a few examples that show the direct cause of rheumatoid arthritis to be food or substances routinely taken into the body. The triggers for this condition are among the most consistent that I have seen in my practice, demonstrating a clear connection on which to base elimination diets. All of these people reported initial complaints involving sore or painful joints, stiffness, and swelling. (These examples will be centered only on arthritic type complaints and not gut dysbiosis.)

Common Triggers
The most common triggers that I have found for the progression of rheumatoid arthritis are dietary, or else a bad habit (such as smoking) that involves the nightshade family and/or gluten. There can be others, like mercury, which can leach from dental fillings; once these amalgams are removed, disease complaints will usually go away systematically. However, all of my treatment cases have primarily involved the diet.

Full Manifestation of Rheumatoid Arthritis Involving Nicotine
I am sharing this case history because I have not come across another like it. The lady was in her early fifties, but with joint malformations that were already very visible. During her appointment, I learned that she didn't eat any of the known culprits for her condition; or, if she did, she did so only rarely. On top of that, she was enviably fit and trim. Even her dental work didn't seem to be a possibility.

However, what she didn't share with me immediately is that she smoked cigarettes. Regardless of how healthy someone appears and claims to be, for joint deformity to occur, something is at the root of this problem. Since tobacco belongs to the nightshade plant family, which has a known scientific reputation for these physical symptoms, my advice to the patient was to quit smoking if she wanted to undo years of tissue damage.

Onset of Rheumatoid Arthritis Involving Gluten
A male in his middle fifties complained about pain and stiffness in his joints. He was diagnosed with the onset of rheumatoid arthritis. His diet was much higher in wheat compared to the nightshade family. He removed gluten from his diet and noticed that the symptoms went away, but, like many people, he tested the waters and was quickly reminded that gluten was the culprit for the onset of his rheumatoid arthritic symptoms.

Thyroiditis and Gluten

In society today, gluten sensitivity is running rampant, with one of its effects being an inflammation of the thyroid gland. Inflammation of the thyroid gland can occur when our immune response goes awry. In such cases, antibodies attack the thyroid gland, causing inflammation. Most people are unaware that gluten has an almost identical matrix to thyroid tissue. Because of this, the immune system does not differentiate between the thyroid gland and the protein gluten, and attacks the thyroid gland simultaneously.

Fibromyalgia

Fibromyalgia is a type of arthritis that manifests as pain, swelling, and stiffness in soft body tissue, ligaments, tendons, and muscles. Fibromyalgia can be very frustrating for patient and doctor alike, since this autoimmune condition may involve any number of symptoms that correlate to several other autoimmune disorders, making a proper diagnosis difficult and time consuming.

In cases such as these, it is imperative to consider treatment protocols that encompass the body as a whole, because there are so many contributing factors to this problem, including:
- Overgrowth of candida
- Leaky gut syndrome
- Low glutathione levels
- Low enzyme activity
- Poor functioning liver
- Imbalanced immune system
- Fibrin over-growth (often due to low protein enzymes)
- Food sensitivities, especially to gluten and nightshade family
- Low serotonin
- Low thyroid function
- Nutrient deficiencies: vitamins, minerals, antioxidant and enzymes
- Infection
- Toxicity
- Poor cellular communication

Fibromyalgia and Gluten
Gluten intolerance is a frequent culprit of fibromyalgia. In my practice, I once worked with a female patient in her fifties, which in itself indicated the possibility of hormonal and endocrine imbalances. She was overweight, with tissue puffiness, slow movement, and had been experiencing pain for many years. The patient consumed high levels of wheat (like pasta, bread, and pastries) and sugar. Her thyroid was low, as were many essential nutrients; in particular, omega-3 fatty acids. For this, I prescribed extra enzymes for digesting protein and instructed her to remove gluten and sugar from her diet.

The challenge with conditions such as this one is that patients can find it difficult to leave their favorite foods alone for long periods. For example, people who love their pasta, especially when it is a major part of their dietary culture, have great difficulty switching to gluten-free. And, once they start to feel much better, they reintroduce the problem element back into their diet—along with their symptom complaints. But is it worth that slice of bread to endure any amount of pain and suffering? It all comes down to choice and discipline.

Fibrin and Proteolytic Enzymes
Fibrin and fibrinogen are produced by the liver to coagulate the blood. This is also the material which forms scar tissue (fibrosis), cysts and other growths. The levels of enzymes that eat up these proteins declines as we age, as part of the natural process. Inadequate live enzyme support through one's diet is another contributing factor.. The consequence of this reduction is an imbalance in the amount of circulating fibrin, which settles throughout the body in glands and tissues.

As fibrosis seeps into our glandular tissue, the levels of hormone production decline. The build-up of scar tissue renders the gland less capable of normal function. As fibrosis weaves its way into our glands, the tissue becomes tough and promotes shrinkage. The end result is premature aging.

When fibrin is the culprit, conditions (of which fibromyalgia could be one) will continue to progress unless measures are taken to remove this substance from the tissues. As a preventive measure and part of a reversal process, diet and nutrient imbalances need to be fully addressed, along with any poor functioning systems such as the endocrine. In cases of fibrin build-up, I recommend a combination formula that includes serrapeptase and proteinase taken on an empty stomach three times a day for six months. These enzymes work systemically and consistently throughout the body to remove fibrin from the muscle tissue.

There are no drugs that can perform this metabolic process; only through the use of properly taken, whole, natural, and effective proteolytic enzymes can scar tissue be removed from the body. Proteolytic enzymes can be purchased in health food stores, as well as online. Once sufficient relief is felt for a protracted period of time, reduce to a maintenance dosage to ensure optimum results. You do not need to continually take these enzymes once the condition clears up, unless you feel a light amount of "insurance" may be valuable.

As a digestive aid, these enzymes are great when taken with a meal including animal protein, especially for the elderly. (Although, be aware that protein consuming enzymes will not work systemically when taken with a meal.) Follow product instructions carefully for best results.

Hypertension May Coincide with Circulating Fibrin
Often when hypertension is an issue, circulation pathways will open up once the fibrin that thickens the blood is lessened or removed. I have witnessed this with patients where, once the pathways opened up, their need for medication for high blood pressure ceased immediately. That said, there may be other circumstances involved with high blood pressure, such as additional chronic illnesses, that cause undue stress on the body's systems and therefore prevents proper functioning. However, for those on high blood pressure medication, monitor your blood pressure closely; for those taking medications that thin the blood, seek professional and medical guidance.

CHAPTER 2

Illnesses Related to Inflammation

So far, medical technology has not been able to keep up with the diet and lifestyle choices being made by the majority of people. Individuals are now being faced with the consequences of excess body fat and long-term, permanent tissue damage. The fact is, when inflammation becomes accelerated and reaches the chronic stage, you have a steady progression towards a shorter life expectancy and prolonged illnesses as the immune system becomes increasingly compromised.

This condition, which has been dubbed "silent inflammation," is simply our immune system responding to various assaults throughout the body. Factors such as obesity, toxicity, and poor dietary and lifestyle habits all contribute to the action and reaction phases of our immune system.

It is only recently that cardiologists have started recognizing that inflammation in the artery wall is the real cause of heart disease, unrelated to elevated blood cholesterol levels. The long-established recommendations for treating heart disease and other chronic illnesses is slowly making a paradigm shift away from traditional therapies, which primarily involved medication.

Let's look at a few of the chronic problems caused by inflammation which continue to affect many North Americans.

Heart Disease

Heart disease continues to top the list of the country's most serious health conditions. According to Johns Hopkins Medicine, statistics show that cardiovascular disease is America's leading health problem *and* the leading cause of death.[6] The American Heart Association recently released num-

---

[6] National Center for Health Statistics, Leading Causes of Death: Centers for Disease Control and Prevention.

bers showing approximately 84 million people have some form of cardiovascular disease, resulting in 2,200 deaths per day—which averages out to one death every forty seconds!

Until recently, the only perceived or recognized cause for heart disease among the allopathic medical community was raised cholesterol levels. Likewise, the only accepted treatment was cholesterol-lowering medications called statins (which twenty-five percent of the population is currently taking), along with drastically lowering one's fat intake. Yet through the abundance of new scientific literature, some heart surgeons are realizing that low fat intake, even when coupled with statins, has not been effective in the prevention of heart related deaths.

One such heart surgeon is Dr. Dwight Lundell, who has performed over 5,000 open heart surgeries and openly admits that the path traditionally taken for the treatment and prevention of this disease has not been a viable solution. Dr. Lundell states, "These recommendations are no longer scientifically or morally defensible." He adds, "It is inflammation that causes cholesterol to become trapped. The injury and inflammation in our blood vessels is caused by the low fat diet recommended for years by mainstream medicine."[7]

Dr. Lundell recognized that without the presence of inflammation, cholesterol could not accumulate in the walls of blood vessels and would therefore flow normally and freely in the body. He now views the inflammatory process to be much the same, regardless of whether it is internal or external. Having seen the inside of thousands of arteries, he describes what a diseased artery looks like: "A diseased artery looks as if someone took a brush and scrubbed repeatedly against its wall. Several times a day, every day, the foods we eat create small injuries compounding into more injuries, causing the body to respond continuously and appropriately with inflammation."[8]

What Food is Causing Inflammation in the Arteries?
The foods and diet imbalances that are shown to produce the most inflammation on the walls of the arteries include:
- Excessive amounts of sugar
- Overabundance of refined carbohydrates
- Flour and their products

7, 8 Dr. Dwight Lundell, "Heart surgeon speaks out on what really causes heart disease." Prevent Disease. March 1, 2012.

- Excess amounts of Omega 6 oils (soybean, vegetable, corn and sunflower)
- Processed foods containing the above mentioned oils

Not surprisingly, these foods have been a main component in the Western diet for decades. The best dietary measure to remove these unwanted fat and calories is by incorporating members of the legume family with each meal containing animal fat or vegetable oils. Beans rate highest for water-soluble fiber, which makes them the ultimate fat grabbers as they bind to fat in the gut. When you eat cooked beans, lentils, or dried peas with a meal, they remove harmful fat substances and old bile acids, all of which are carried out in your fecal matter. In this way, the body is forced to produce new, stronger bile that further enhances cholesterol removal throughout the body, including the arteries.

Generally, I recommend one-quarter to one-half cup of beans per meal containing animal fat or vegetable oils. If you are a candidate for heart disease, do this for six months to one year, while remembering to incorporate beans into your general diet as a preventive measure and weight loss aid.

> For a complete guide on heart disease reversal processes and related conditions, pick up the previous book in this series, *Reverse Heart Disease Naturally*. It contains the latest scientifically-backed supplements for lowering cholesterol and high blood pressure (without medication), as well as super-nutrients to boost weakened hearts, correct fatigue, and support a low functioning body. *Reverse Heart Disease Naturally* also contains an excellent step-by-step diet program to help you reach your optimum cardiovascular health, with the side benefit of steady weight loss for those who desire it. Remember, no matter your age, heart disease is reversible and preventable.

Cancer

The factors involved in developing a tumor are very complex. Nonetheless, we know that inflammation is the driving force in a cancer's development, all aspects of its growth, and its spread throughout the body. The link between cancer and inflammation was first discovered by Rhudolf

Virchow, a German pathologist, who was also the first person to discover immune cells existing in cancer tumors.[9] He then made the correlation between inflammation and tumors, which has continued on in present day research.

Angiogenesis
A tumor requires the same elements for survival as any other main body part (such as an organ). It needs a support system of blood vessels to supply itself with nutrition, oxygen, and waste removal. Tumors use a process called angiogenesis, which describes how a tumor draws its blood supply from nearby blood vessels. The angiogenesis process is one of great interest to researchers all over the world, as it is the primary means for how cancer manifests and spreads in the body.

At the outset, a minuscule tumor can gather enough nutrition and oxygen from its surrounding environment. But things quickly become desperate when the tumor's ecosystem can no longer support its growth. At this point, the tumor is forced to go further afield for what it needs, which draws more attention from the immune system. The tumor, in its struggle to survive, sends out malfunctioning signals that attract immune cells (macrophages and granulocytes), which penetrate the tumor. Upon entering the tumor, these immune cells begin secreting cytokines, which now induces angiogenesis (growth of new blood vessels). Once oxygen and nutrition is supplied to the tumor, it continues to establish itself through various cytokines. Certain cytokines prepare the area where the tumor will rest (called the stroma) by initiating cellular growth to cushion and support its mass.

Meanwhile, free radicals (such as inflammatory cells) are sprayed onto the tumor, which causes further DNA impairment. Research has suggested that inflammation could also be what promotes spreading of the tumor. By picturing this series of events, it's not hard to imagine how immature tumors use the inflammation process to accelerate into a full blown disease like cancer.

For some time now, drug companies have been trying to find a way in which to manipulate inflammation in an attempt to try and prevent the onset and spread of cancer. It has even been suggested that taking aspirin

---

9 Rudolph Virchow. Theory on cancer origin: Wagner, RP (1999). "Anecdotal, historical and critical commentaries on genetics. Rudolph Virchow and the genetic basis of somatic ecology". Genetics. 151 (3): 917–920. PMID 10049910.

may be a solution, since it dampens inflammation. But aspirin, just like all the other medications, comes with its own list of shortcomings.

Problems such as cancer develop over long periods of time. Regardless of inflammation's role in the process, an environment was first set up to allow for rogue cells to mature and proliferate. Evaluate your diet and determine what areas may need to be adjusted. Chapter 10 contains great dietary guidance that will help rebalance and change your internal environment while strengthening your overall immune system.

Diabetes

Looking at human history, obesity is a newcomer to the human condition. Therefore, it should be no surprise that evolution has ill-equipped us to handle the imbalances produced by an overload of adipose tissue. The relationship between diabetes and inflammation has been documented for over one hundred years. The discovery was first recognized when it was observed that the application of high doses of salycilates (an anti-inflammatory) caused symptoms of type 2 diabetes to go away.

Inflammation is known to precede insulin resistance and (possibly) obesity. There is also a very close association between obesity and diabetes. When taking a closer look at our fat cells, many would be surprised to learn that our adipose tissue contains many hormones and is an active part of our physiology. Naturally, as a person becomes obese, their fat cells are initially affected. One of the ways research has indicated that inflammation sets the stage for obesity and type 2 diabetes is through the effect initiated by elevated levels of inflammatory cytokines upon healthy, normal cells, producing insulin resistance.

For every twenty pounds of extra body weight, there is a significant and measurable inflammation response brought on by your own immune system. It is therefore highly recommended to maintain a healthy body weight in order prevent the many chronic conditions associated with prolonged inflammation.

Obesity
As noted, an overall contributor for setting up the body for inflammation is obesity. Many Americans are struggling with excess belly fat, but are unaware of how this type of fat storage affects inflammation, especially in women. It is a virtual engine of inflammation! The inflammation chemicals TNF-alpha (Eur J Endocrinal 2001) has shown to be significantly

higher in obese women as well as obese children (J Prediatr Endocrinol 2001). While overweight people in general, in particular those with excess belly weight, face another dangerous chemical (inflammation compound IL-6) showing to be higher in these individuals.

Insulin Resistance and Inflammation
Researchers have been on the hunt for reasons why fat tissue spurs chronic inflammation. In particular, they have been examining cytokine signaling and macrophage behavior; as the fat mass expands, additional stress at a cellular level may lead to the dysfunction of our main energy source, the mitochondria. Another influence upon the cells may be oxidative stress. As more glucose becomes available to the fat cells, they manufacture an excess of reactive oxygen species (ROS), which begins an inflammatory cycle in the cells.

An initiating source of insulin resistance is the secretion of inflammatory cytokines, TFN-a (Tumor Necrosis Factor-alpha) and Interleukin-6 (IL-6), which are released during inflammation, as well as MCP-1 and C-reactive proteins. TFN-a is a cell signaling protein, and is one of the cytokines that participates in acute phase inflammation reactions. It also has a role in systemic inflammation. The cytokine Interleukin-6 is involved in inflammation and infections, as well as the regulatory functions of regenerative, metabolic, and neural systems. Monocyte Chemoattractant Protein (MCP1) is a chemokine, also referred to as monocyte chemotactic protein 1 (MCP1) and small cytokine A2. C-reactive protein (CRP) is a blood test marker for inflammation in the body (produced in the liver) which will rise in response to inflammation.

Due to the increased levels of the white cells called macrophages, these immune cells gather in the fat cells, which incites a release of the aforementioned inflammatory cytokines.

Leptin Hormone
There is a direct connection between inflammation of the hypothalamus (referred to as "the appetite center of the brain") and excess body fat, as well as insulin resistance and energy expenditure. This connection comes about through our fat cells, via the hormone leptin. When the body is functioning properly, leptin helps to inhibit and regulate hunger, as well as energy balance, glycemia and neuroendocrine functions. Released from fat cells in the adipose tissue, leptin sends signals to the hypothalamus that dictate a feeling of satiety, or feeling full.

Ideally, when excess fat cells produce leptin, the hypothalamus is stimulated to lower one's appetite, thereby encouraging the body to burn up its fat stores for more energy. However, when there is too much body fat, there is in turn too much leptin, which impairs the hypothalamus' ability to balance energy output effectively. This is because obesity impairs leptin signaling, desensitizes its physiological responses and causes leptin resistance.

In addition, glucose metabolism becomes impaired by insulin and leptin resistance. The consequence is hyperglycemia, a condition in which fat cells can no longer store any more glucose; the cells themselves have become insulin resistant. This process leads to further inflammation in the form of advanced glycation endproducts (AGEs), many of which are connected to type-2 diabetes.

Autism

Autism has increased tenfold in the last twenty years. Despite many years of assuming that autism is primarily a brain disorder, many children are now seeing improvement through treating the biological imbalances involved in the condition, rather than treating its resulting behaviors.

Although autism is described as a complex neurological disorder, in recent scientific trials researchers have identified in autistic patients nearly double the normal levels of oxidative stress as a result of excessive free radicals. Because of this enhanced production of free radicals, we see an increase in the imbalance of the body's main antioxidant defense system. Our brain cells are highly susceptible to damage from free radicals; the young brains of developing children are at higher risk.

Normally, our brain cells are protected by the antioxidant glutathione, which is (hopefully) found in every cell in our body and which serves as our liver's main antioxidant. Autistic children, by contrast, have been diagnosed with brain inflammation and high levels of toxic metals, while exhibiting low levels of glutathione, zinc, metallothionein (MT) and sulfur. Additionally, poorly-functioning digestive systems (including leaky gut), as well as allergies, amino acid imbalances, and protein absorption problems, further compound their inflammation and their resulting behavioral issues.

Because of these low antioxidant levels, children with autism are less able to detoxify heavy metals found in the air, chemicals in their food, and vaccine preservatives like aluminum and thimerosal.

A research team led by Dr. Domenico Pratico, an associate professor of

Pharmacology, published the results of their autism study in the August 2006 issue of the Archives of Neurology. Their findings revealed that the rate of thromboxane (an index of platelet activation) and prostacyclin synthesis (a measure of blood vessel activation) both showed to be significantly increased in autistic children. These conditions are closely correlated with the production rate of oxidative stress. The reports states, "Children with autism have significantly higher urinary levels of isoprostane, thromboxane, and prostacyclin."[10]

Dr. Alexander Schauss, known for his excellent work with plant antioxidants such as anthocyanins, commented on the above study in reference to reducing oxidative stress. He suggests that by consuming quality juices that contain high levels of antioxidants, a reduction of oxidative stress and improvement of blood vessel function may be possible. Examples of suitably high quality juices include those from berries such as acai, aronia, wolfberry and wild blueberries, which has shown results in the treatment of patients with autism and ADHD, and even Tourette's syndrome and seizures.

Brain Inflammation and Autism

Dr. Herbert, a Harvard pediatric neurologist, knew he'd discovered something important when, while observing the white matter of the brain, he had an epiphany: "Could white matter become chronically inflamed?"

Supportive research was provided by Carlos Pardo, a neurologist at Johns Hopkins, in a 2005 study in the Annals of Neurology, where he found inflammation in immune responsive brain cells of autistic patients. Dr. Pardo states, "Patients with autism report lots of immunological problems. We looked for the fingerprints of those problems in the brain. We had brain tissue from autistic individuals as young as 5 and as old as 45 and we found neuroglia inflammation in all of them. Neuroglia is a group of brain cells that are important in the brain's immune response. This inflammatory reaction appears to happen both early and late in the course of the disorder. If it happens early, it could dramatically influence brain development. We're very excited about this research because one potential treatment approach then, is to down regulate the brain's immune response."

---

10 Pratico D, Lawson JA, Rokach J, FitzGerald GA. The isoprostanes in biology and medicine. Trends Endor Metabol. 2001;12:243-247

Treating Autism with Flavonoids
When considering methods of treating and preventing inflammation through natural means, few options have the wealth of benefits available that consuming flavonoids represents. From mild protective benefits to actively fighting degenerative diseases, noticeable improvements have been shown in the following areas after regular consumption of flavonoids: reduced inflammation; fewer epileptic seizures; improved behavior; increased mental clarity; and better relationship interactions. The highest antioxidant levels are typically found in fruits and berries native to the hottest regions of the world. They possess far greater amounts of these special flavonoids compared to foods consumed in the northern hemisphere, because they act as the plant's sunscreen in nature. Examples of such fruits, presented in sequence of antioxidant level, are as follows: acai, aronia, pomegranates, cranberries, cherries and blueberries. A double blind study revealed that when participants consumed four ounces of juice made from berries possessing high levels of antioxidants, their antioxidant levels increased by 82 percent compared to the placebo group (AIBMR Life Sciences Inc. Natural and Medicinal products research).

High-quality juice products can be purchased in a variety of stores and through direct sales companies. To ensure the highest quality possible when purchasing products from great distances, buy only those that have been processed with a flash frozen, freeze-dried method. Most companies use a heat-dried method, which significantly reduces the oxygen radical absorption capacity (ORAC). (Note as well that if your berry of choice is the acai, be certain to investigate the processing method before you buy. Most of the acai products currently being sold have removed the very valuable essential fatty acids.)

Metabolic Syndrome

Metabolic syndrome (METs) is a relatively new category in medicine that has been shown to predict diabetes and heart attacks in adults and adolescents. Indicators for the syndrome consist of a collection of imbalances that, when they all come together, form the diagnosis of metabolic syndrome.

The indicators for metabolic syndrome mainly consist of the following risk factors:
- High blood pressure and high triglyceride levels, accompanied by low HDL (good cholesterol levels)
- Insulin resistance, allowing for an excess of glucose in the blood supply due to faulty functioning of normal insulin levels
- Elevated levels of inflammation markers TNF-alpha, interleukin 6, and CRP
- Fat distribution in the stomach and lower abdomen (android fat)

Inflammation markers are involved in all aspects of this syndrome, and are therefore implicated in the development of metabolic syndrome. Several studies have suggested that a pro-inflammatory state is one factor of metabolic syndrome, as well as accumulating evidence revealing that low-grade inflammation is associated with endothelial dysfunction.

Effects of Diet on Metabolic Syndrome
In looking to determine the possible effects of diet on metabolic syndrome, Mediterranean diet patients were given a program for increasing their daily consumption of whole grains, fruits, vegetables, nuts, and olive oil. Following the two-year study, those with the greatest improvement also had a lower ratio intake of omega 6 pro-inflammatory fatty acids, compared to anti-inflammatory omega 3 fatty acids. They also experienced more weight loss and a greater increase of energy.

The results of the Mediterranean diet proved successful, with patients showing a reduction in many components of their metabolic syndrome; so much so that the overall prevalence of this syndrome was reduced by half. A few notable results included significantly reduced serum concentration of CRP levels and inflammation markers, as well as decreased insulin resistance. Patients also displayed improvements in their endothelial function and a significant reduction of indicators of systemic vascular inflammation.[11]

The DASH diet (Dietary Approaches to Stop Hypertension) has also been examined to determine its effects on patients with metabolic syn-

---
11 Katherine Esposito, MD; Raffaele Marfella MD, PhD. Effect of a Mediterranean-Style Diet on Endothelial Dysfunction and Markers of Vascular Inflammation in the Metabolic Syndrome. September 22/29, 2004.

drome. Comparable to other healthy routines, the program involves a lower calorie intake, while increasing fruits and vegetables (four to six per day), whole grains and legumes, and low-fat dairy, while also decreasing saturated fat, salt and cholesterol. A trial event involving 116 outpatients (divided into three groups) on a controlled diet for six months demonstrated the value of eating more fruits and vegetables. They exhibited the following benefits: an increase in good cholesterol (HDL); reduced blood pressure; lower blood glucose levels; and weight loss. In addition, only 65 percent of the participants continued to suffer with METs once the trial had finished.[12]

Asthma, Allergy and Sinusitis

A constant problem among children and adults throughout the world are the symptoms associated with asthma, allergies, and sinus conditions. Inflammation is well marked in all of these illnesses. Yet as annoying as these problems are, simple diet changes and additions can bring about noticeable improvements. A study using the Mediterranean diet involving 690 children ages 7–18 showed that those children who consumed grapes more often had lower incidence of wheezing, while those who ate more kiwi and oranges experienced fewer sinus problems. Interestingly, Greece is a part of the world that reports very few allergies. Most feel this is due to their omega-3 rich diet, abundant in fresh fish. The Mediterranean diet is also very rich in antioxidants, derived from fresh salads, olives, onions, and tomatoes.

There are also vitamins and minerals known to directly affect the nasal passageways. For instance, a lack of vitamin A is a main contributor to sinusitis, while the mineral selenium may be used to help ward off asthma attacks. By introducing beta-carotene rich foods (orange, red and yellow fruits and vegetables), patients have seen a reduction in inflammation and reduced symptoms. Apple peels contain allergy and inflammation fighting flavonoids such as quercetin, catechin, epicatechin, and procyanidins. (Quercetin is often taken as a supplement at the onset of allergy symptoms and, at times, for allergy related hives).

---

12 Leila Azadbakht, MSC, Parvin Mirmiran, MSC, Ahmad Esmaillzadeh, MSC, Tohid Azizi, MD and Fereidoun Azizi, MD + Author Affiliations. From the Endocrine Research Center, Shaheed Beheshti University of Medical Sciences, Tehran, Iran

Reducing Mucus through Diet
The problem of thick, annoying mucus is not restricted to just those with chronic sinus and allergy conditions. People who consume high amounts of sugar, dairy and starchy carbohydrates often experience a constant mucus presence. But by simply eliminating mucus-forming foods like ice cream, patients have seen an amazing reduction in mucus-related symptoms. Apple cider vinegar, on the other hand, thins the mucus in your body so it can flow out through the bowels rather than accumulating in the throat and sinuses. Adding a tablespoon of apple cider vinegar to a small amount of water and drinking one to three times a day will show noticeable improvement. Follow this with a light maintenance program that will keep things moving and significantly reduce mucus forming from the foods you consume.

Saline irrigation is another great tool for targeting and decreasing nasal congestion. It works better than nasal sprays. Nasal irrigation pots are easily purchased at pharmacies. When purchasing saline solution, make sure it does not contain the preservative benzalkonium, as this chemical can impair nasal function and may sting and burn. To make your own, simply add one teaspoon of a quality salt (like Himalayan salt) to 500 ml of distilled water.

Boosting the Immune System
An ideal way to prevent sinus issues and other infections is to create an inhospitable environment. Maintaining a robust immune system will drastically reduce the onset of colds, which are the number one trigger for inflammation of the mucous membranes. Be sure to include immune-boosting foods and supplements in your diet, such as omega 3 fish oil, probiotics, vitamins C and D, and the minerals zinc and iodine. (In fact, iodine has been noted since the early 1900s for destroying influenza. Today, iodine is recognized for being a virus, mold, yeast and bacteria fighter, destroying most bacterium within 25–30 seconds of contact.)

Consider using coconut oil for cooking; it is less toxic to heat and contains lauric acid, which possesses antiviral, antibacterial, and antifungal properties.

The next chapter will take you through the inflammatory pathways that are directly affected by dietary fats. You will also learn about the worst contributors and instigators for enhancing inflammation, and ways to block or inhibit these culprits.

CHAPTER 3

Key Players of the Inflammatory Response

OUR BODIES ARE not designed to process foods that are laden with sugar and drenched in oils. The vicious cycle of consuming poor fats and mountains of sugar leads to a laundry list of conditions, including diabetes, heart disease, hypertension, dementia, autoimmune disease, metabolic syndrome, and cancer.

Not surprisingly, when the word "vegetable" or "natural" is attached to an item, the general impression is usually that the item is healthy. Unfortunately, death by vegetable oil is more likely than people might think. During the 20th century, household consumption and food industry usage of vegetable oil has dramatically risen, with devastating results. The problem has to do with how these oils are manufactured, as well as their high toxicity, which cripples our immune system.

The supposedly "healthy" oils—those labeled polyunsaturated—are among the worst offenders for inflammation. In fact, saturated animal fat is far less likely to cause inflammation. Bear in mind that processed foods most often contain soybean and corn oil. Their concentration of omega-6 fatty acids is very high, while not containing any omega-3 fatty acids. Our body's physiology dictates the proper ratio of omega-6 verses omega-3 fatty acids for health and longevity.

PERCENTAGE OF OMEGA 6 COMPARED TO OMEGA 3		
1 tablespoon =	Omega 6	Omega 3
Corn oil	7,280 mg	0 mg
Soybean oil	6,940 mg	0 mg
Sunflower oil	10,602 mg	0 mg
Safflower oil	10,073 mg	0 mg
Olive oil	1318 mg	103 mg
Flaxseed oil	1715 mg	7196 mg
Fish oil	0 mg	100 percent

Omega-3 EFAs

There are major differences between omega-3 and omega-6 fatty acids, even though they seem to share the same identity. The most striking difference is how they perform in our bodies. Omega-3 fats, derived from fish and seeds, are the primary fats necessary for all body functions and cell growth and restoration. Recent advancements made by scientists and researchers have shown that these essential fats are required everywhere in the body. This, by inverse, means that a lack of omega-3s—coupled with an imbalance of other dietary fats—is one of the main instigators for disease.

The omega-3 fatty acids found in fish oil contain docosahexaenoic acid (DHA) and eicosapentaenoic acid (EPA). These special elements have been shown to benefit many heart-related problems when consumed in appropriate dosages. A few examples are lower triglyceride levels, suppler arteries, stroke prevention, normalization of heart arrhythmias, lower blood pressure, and less sticky blood (which improves circulation).

Another essential fatty acid related to omega-3s is alpha-linolenic acid (ALA). Higher sources of ALAs include seeds and nuts, as well as certain spices and vegetables, but these are short chain-fatty acids (as compared to long chain-fatty acids, found in their highest quantities in fish, seafood and fish oil products). This is an important fact, since only long-chained fatty acids can feed the brain directly and efficiently.

Vegetarians must get their EPA and DHA from vegetarian sourced ALAs, through the conversion of these fats by the body. The short chained alpha linolenic acid (ALA) found in plants may be difficult to convert to DHA. There is some controversy over whether or not this process is always successful, since it is slow and perhaps incomplete. To help ensure the availability of sufficient levels of long chain fatty acids, the recommended dosage is 4:1, or 4 parts omega-3s (such as chia and flax oil) to 1 part omega-6 fatty acids (found in olive and vegetable oils). I have had vegetarian/vegan patients who had to reintroduce fish oils because they were becoming unwell.

The list of duties performed by omega-3 fatty acids is extensive, but for our purposes, they fight inflammation throughout the body and are particularly important for brain health. The following are a few more reasons to make omega 3s part of your daily routine.

- Inflammation response requires an omega-3 fatty acid
- Immune response also requires an omega-3 fatty acid
- Nerve communication could not occur in a normal way without these fats
- Core component in the spinal cord, sensory glands, brain and nervous system
- Brain mass consists of over 60 percent long chain fatty acids
- Needed for proper retinal and brain development
- Liver needs omega-3 fatty acids for proper cholesterol balancing
- Cell membranes utilize omega 3 fats in their construction
- Necessary role in hormone production
- Preserves blood levels of vitamin D
- Keeps the blood smooth and non-sticky

Once you become aware of the significance of omega-3 fatty acids in the diet and their role in the human body, you will quickly form a picture as to the reasons why you feel as you do.

The Problem with Omega-6 EFAs
A major issue involved in having consistently high levels of omega-6 in your diet is that it creates a deficiency of omega-3, as both of these fats compete for the same converting enzymes in the body. Thankfully, the reverse is true; with sufficient stores of omega-3 fatty acids, the inflammation promoting omega-6 cannot compete for conversion of alpha linoleic acid for eicosanoid production.

> **Eicosanoid Processes**
>
> Biochemically, eicosanoids are signaling molecules made by the oxidation of fatty acids (both omega-3 and omega-6 fatty acids). They employ multifaceted control over many systems and are very complex in their duties throughout the body. Eicosanoids control inflammation and immunity when the body has been threatened, as well as serve as the carrier for messages via the central nervous system.
>
> Omega-6 eicosanoids are pro-inflammatory, while omega-3 fatty acids protect against inflammation and disease. Ultimately, the balance of omega-6 verses omega-3 fats in ones diet will affect the body's eicosanoid-controlled functions.
>
> As a side note, over-the-counter and prescription medications designed to reduce the inflammatory mechanisms derive their function from these pathways. In essence, NSAIDs reduce inflammation by artificially inhibiting the eicosanoid pathways. Therefore, by really focusing on the reduction of your dietary intake of omega-6 fats, you can achieve the same effect. (For additional benefit and quicker results, increase your omega-3 based fats, since inflammation response does require an omega-3 fatty acid.)

The sad truth is that most people's diets are between a ratio of 20–30 to 1 of omega-6 fats compared to omega-3 fats. Besides the obvious sources for omega-6 fats being fast food, processed food, junk food, and eating out, it is also a main element in many households' everyday cooking. The majority of the population has grown up cooking with vegetable or peanut oil (and, to a lesser degree, olive oil).

For the most part, the average person is uneducated on the processes involved in oil production. Most of us have misplaced our trust in government agencies, thinking our families are protected by those who regulate and control food and drugs. Fortunately, with the help of global media, more awareness on the ills and misconceptions about how our food is grown, its quality, and the toxicity it may contain has become available—if you know how to look for it.

In searching for the truth about your cooking oils, you might ask yourself: "Is my olive oil really pure extra virgin? Is my vegetable oil GMO-based and chemical-laden?" We'll therefore start with the process for making these oils and their effect on the human body.

Oil Production Process

A disturbing fact is that the majority of vegetable oil contains industrialized chemicals and extremely toxic solvents, and is processed to the point of being foodless. These processes lessen acid content but add toxic vapors, pesticides, and enzymes and proteins that are sourced from genetically modified organisms (GMOs).

In learning the ins and outs for how omega-6-based oils are processed in the body, you may have come to realize that overconsumption of vegetable oil will cause structural change in our cells and an imbalance in our fat stores. Oils that are sourced from genetically modified plants confuse our cells, destroying our defenses and (in some cases) damaging the mitochondria in our cells. Oils associated with GMOs include sunflower, soybean, corn, canola, safflower and cottonseed. Persistent and excessive use of such oils will lead directly to multiple illnesses and symptom complaints.

Grapeseed Oil Process
The process for extracting oil from grape seeds is even more distressing. A hydrocarbon called hexane, which is a main component of gasoline, and inexpensive solvents typically used in the manufacturing of glue for textiles, footwear, roofing, and much more, is used to extract oil from seeds. Thankfully, cold pressed (hexane-free) grape seed oil is available.

Rapeseed (Canola) Oil
The history of rapeseed oil is a bit sketchy. It was banned in the U.S. in the fifties and resurfaced only after a Canadian scientist made it less toxic—which does not indicate that it is now a healthy choice. Rapeseed oil—better known as canola oil—is 90 percent partially hydrogenated and, like most other oils, is a GMO product. Canola oil is widely used in the food industry, especially in restaurants and grocery stores.

Olive Oil
Disappointingly, more than half of the olive oil sold in North America is not pure or extra virgin. Apparently, these oils (referred to as hybrids) are a mixture of toxic canola oil (rapeseed), GMO soybean oil, and other sub-grade oils.

Coconut Oil

These issues don't seem to apply to organic coconut oil. More and more of my patients are informing me that they use coconut oil for cooking without ill effects, so it may be that coconut oil can provide an answer to this oil madness.

Free Radicals Affect Disease and Inflammation

A free radical is an unstable molecule that steals electrons from other healthy cells in an attempt to stabilize itself. When this occurrence becomes repetitive, we experience damage to our cells, protein molecules, and DNA as a consequence of their chemical structure being altered. In other words, free radicals can take normal elements in the body and co-opt them for themselves, creating something in the process which the body may not be prepared to deal with.

Free radicals occupy our day-to-day space in the form of industrial contaminants, metal toxicity, toxic products, and cigarette smoke, as well as pollutants such as herbicides, pesticides, and insecticides. Free radicals have been shown to initiate the disease and inflammation process, and can cause oxidative stress linked to a wide variety of problems, including chronic inflammation, Alzheimer's, Parkinson's, diabetes, heart disease, neurological problems, cancer, arthritic conditions, incidences of pain, and much more.

Free radicals *can* be beneficial when in the form of a byproduct that is consistent with a natural metabolic process, but not when it's introduced from an outside source. In today's industrialized environment, with today's poor dietary habits, we now have an optimal setting for destructive free radicals. Free radicals and inflammation are also induced by elevated levels of microbes and pathogens such as parasites, fungus, yeast, bacteria and viruses, plus vaccines and medications. Our bodies become susceptible to free radicals through a lack of dietary vitamins and minerals, antioxidants, amino acids, and enzymes.

Free Radicals and Antioxidants

Our immune system makes a great effort to ward off free radicals through naturally manufactured antioxidants in the body. Most times, this attempt will fall short unless the body is supported with live, whole foods and quality antioxidant supplementation. Antioxidants will be fully described in

Chapter 5, including detailed sources and applications. For now, let's take a quick look at how they support the body against free radical damage.

An antioxidant, at the basic level, is a molecule that defends or slows down the oxidation of other molecules. Antioxidants generously offer up their electrons to free radicals for stabilization to prevent tissue and cellular damage. However, each time an antioxidant neutralizes a free radical by sacrificing its electrons, it then stops being able to function as an antioxidant. Herein lies the great value of consuming concentrated nutrients found in raw juices, as well as those fruits and vegetables containing exceptionally high levels of antioxidants. Antioxidants are our first and best line of defense against inflammation and many degenerative diseases.

Candida Causes Inflammation

The distinction has been made that inflammation is not at the root of all disease, and that rather a cause must be in place for it to persist; otherwise, it is a natural, healthy immune response. When an area of the body becomes damaged or is deteriorating, inflammation becomes either a temporary or a permanent fixture.

Several causes have already been explored, and there will be more to come, but one of the roots for disease is an overgrowth of candida albicans that has made its way into the lining of our intestinal tract, causing gut permeability. When our intestinal lining becomes compromised, it allows for unwanted proteins, particles, sugar molecules, and bacteria to seep into the bloodstream. This will automatically initiate an immune response causing inflammation. These and other pathogens also release toxic substances throughout their life cycle, known for degrading and decaying tissues within the gastrointestinal tract.

Candida seems to be more of a permanent fixture since it appears to be much hardier than other bacteria. It is an opportunistic pathogen that flourishes when the good gut flora (acidophilus and bifidus strains, also known as probiotics) becomes insufficient in our intestinal tract. Another element that alters the balance of the friendly flora in our body are toxic chemicals and genetically modified organisms (GMOs). Pesticide and GMO-laden foods all have an adverse effect on our good gut bacteria. Candida will once again bounce back (as will other pathogens) as toxins continue to invade the intestinal tract.

Recommendations for Combating Candida
The single greatest cause for the proliferation of candida is the misuse of antibiotics. Familiarize yourself with the safe and effective natural anti-viral and anti-bacterial replacements for antibiotics. These products can be found in whole food and health-oriented stores in combination formulas or as singular preparations. A few excellent choices are colloidal silver, oregano oil, turmeric (curcumin), Manuka honey, and Sutherlandia frutescens.

That said, the quickest way to reduce candida and microbes in the intestinal tract is by cutting off their food supply and rebuilding the integrity of the gut flora. Whether it is fungus, yeast, or other bacteria, sugar is a main contributor to most infectious microorganisms. Nearly all forms of sugar and refined carbohydrates, such as white flour products, pasta, and rice, need to be removed from your diet, as these items and similar ones feed the undesirable life forms in our gut.

For more aggressive elimination of candida, caprylic acid is a plant substance with strong antifungal properties and a proven track record for eliminating yeast overgrowth. Take as suggested for one month to pick up all the stages of microbial growth, while following dietary restrictions for sugar and sugar producing foods. When purchasing caprylic acid, be sure to buy full strength; the dosage amount contained in combination formulas may not be high enough.

As a last note, citrus seed extract and garlic are two other effective agents to fight yeast and fungus, and black walnut hull extract is especially good for fungus and parasites. I routinely use these extracts when treating all manners of yeast-related illnesses, including cystitis, bladder infection, candidiasis, *H. pylori*, systemic fungus infection, and certain skin disorders.

When the goal is disease reversal, it is important to address all main areas of the body, as large gaps in nutrition ultimately lead to chronic imbalance. Inflammation is always a by-product, but the nutrients that help balance the inflammatory pathways in the body are also the ones most required for health maintenance and disease prevention.

What we eat will always play a key role in our health and well-being. Therefore, we will now take a look at commonly eaten foods that add to or initiate the inflammation process, as well as discussing the harmful chemicals contained in and around our food that can harm the cells in our bodies and incite inflammation.

CHAPTER 4

Foods and Substances that Trigger Inflammation

THE KEY TO reducing inflammation in your body starts with the diet. By familiarizing yourself with specific foods that have shown a propensity for triggering inflammation, you will reduce your risk of chronic disease and live a more pain-free life.

While it may seem like common sense, the foods that are most likely causing your discomfort are the ones that you most routinely take into your body. The majority of mainstream complaints related to diet often starts out as food sensitivity and build into intolerance.

But is it actually the food that's causing the problem?

For example, consider celiac disease. In cases of celiac, there will be antibodies that show up in a blood test to indicate an intolerance or allergy to the protein gluten. However, there are plenty of individuals who become gluten sensitive because of gut permeability and leaky gut, whether through use of antibiotics, anti-inflammatory medications, or prolonged usage of over-the-counter painkillers. At the same time, their leaky gut may be caused by bad habits like cigarettes and alcohol abuse, or acid- and chemically-laden beverages such as coffee and soda.

Whatever the reason, the body is responding to an alarm signal, which sets in motion a series of immune processes that will either deal with the situation or further lead to chronic inflammation and tissue damage. The point is, our diet is affected by our lifestyle, and reversing a person's chronic inflammation may require more than just increased supplementation or an elimination diet.

Foods to Avoid

Pro-inflammatory foods and substances help inflammation take root in your body, and have a direct influence on the severity of your inflammation. Unfortunately, the standard American diet is teeming with highly processed foods that are loaded with preservatives, chemical additives, bad fats and sugar. Depending on your diet, you can affect a chain of events that can actually stimulate or worsen the inflammation process.

Be on the alert for the following foods and substances to reduce the effects of inflammation and prevent further tissue damage.

Fried Foods: Foods that are fried, charred, or barbecued are not only inflammatory, but carcinogenic as well. When foods are cooked at high heat or burnt, it incites an inflammatory response due to the process of advanced glycation end products (AGEs). AGEs are created when a protein is bound to a glucose molecule. This results in damaged cross-linked proteins. The body's natural immune response kicks into action and secretes large amounts of cytokines in an attempt to break apart these proteins.

It is interesting to note that many diseases involved with aging are actually part of this process. Depending on where the body's immune response takes place, it can lead to conditions of heart disease, arthritis, cataracts, diabetes, dementia, and premature aging.

Sugar: Avoid all refined white sugar, corn syrup, candy, and products made from these sugars.

Refined White Flour: There are important reasons for eliminating all refined white flour and their products from your diet, besides the fact that it is "foodless" food. Our digestive process starts in the mouth, where starches and sugars are initially broken down by our saliva. Starch products become sugar molecules that are quickly absorbed, which then spikes your blood sugar. When blood sugar spikes, so does inflammation.

White flour is also akin to wallpaper paste in our gut—it's very difficult for the body to move it along. Many people are instead opting for gluten-free grains and products for their easier digestibility, lower calories, and higher nutritional value.

Red and Processed Meat: Eliminate the following protein sources when inflammation is present: beef, pork, hot dogs, cold cuts, sausages, and shellfish. While red meat may not be the culprit of chronic inflammation; rather, it may be due to an imbalance of the omega-3 fatty acids, accompanied by higher levels of omega-6 oils and carbohydrates. Regardless, eliminating red and processed meat can serve to reduce inflammation symptoms.

Eggs: If you have an intolerance for or a digestion problem with eggs, it would be advisable to leave them alone.

Dairy: When inflammation is a concern, avoid all cows' milk products, including milk, cream, yogurt, butter and ice cream. It's common knowledge that we no longer have the enzyme for digesting lactose after the age of 3 years; it is only because we have continued to consume the product for centuries that individuals find they can tolerate the protein casein and the milk sugar lactose.

Nightshade Plant Family: Avoid tomatoes, eggplant, peppers (bell), chilies (hot), tomatillo, gooseberry, Goji berry, and tobacco. Refer to Chapter 1 for more information about nightshade's properties and the inflammation problems associated with this plant species.

Gluten: Grains and seitan, including wheat gluten, mock duck, and wheat meat, should be avoided. Refer to Chapter 1 for conditions related to gluten sensitivity.

Wheat: Amylopectin is a property found in wheat shown to spike blood sugar more than table sugar. It may also be a sensitivity or intolerant among celiac patients.

Grains: Whether you are gluten sensitive or not, grains such as wheat, corn, barley, rye, kamut, and spelt heighten inflammation in the body.

Soy: Remove all soy products, including tempeh, tofu, soymilk, soy protein substitute, and dehydrated soy products.

Corn and Processed Corn: Similar to gluten, not everyone will have a problem digesting corn. For those that are sensitive to gluten, corn may trigger an immune response. However, when it comes to processed corn products, there are several derivatives known for increasing inflammation and raising blood sugar levels. Because it is cheap and subsidized by the government, products like corn syrup and corn oil are used everywhere. Read labels to avoid these items (cornstarch can be replaced with arrowroot and tapioca powder).

Nuts: Peanuts and peanut butter have been shown to increase inflammation.

Oranges: In cases of acid reflux or gastric ulcers, adding oranges to your diet can produce increased inflammation and nausea.

Beverages: Reduce and eliminate all acidic liquids, including coffee, black tea, soda, diet soft drinks, caffeinated beverages, and alcohol. Highly acidic and irritating properties cause gut permeability and adversely affect our good gut flora (acidophilus and bifidus).

Condiments: If inflammation is a real concern, remove these and similar items from your diet: ketchup, mustard, chocolate, relish, chutney, barbecue sauce, and soy sauce.

Oils: The following oils are known contributors to inflammation throughout the body: canola (rapeseed), cottonseed, palm, sunflower, safflower, grapeseed (except cold-pressed), peanut, and fake olive oil.

Commercial products: Margarine, shortening, commercial spreads, mayonnaise, and other hydrogenated oil based food products have all been shown to heighten inflammation.

Microwave popcorn: Inflammation is linked to the artificial butter and the bag itself (in most popcorn brands). These products contain hydrogenated oils (trans fats) and the fumes given off from the steaming bag contain a lung irritant.

There are wonderful air popping machines for the weight conscious individual, or you can make it the traditional way on the stove. Otherwise, for a healthier approach to using the microwave, put one-quarter to one-third cup of corn kernels into a brown paper bag and microwave for two minutes or until the corn stops popping.

Inflammation-Causing Chemicals

Chemicals have become a permanent fixture in our environment and diet. In order to ensure that you have all the information necessary to combat inflammation, you must understand the roles that these artificial substances play when we take them into our bodies.

Artificial Sweeteners
Besides the lengthy list of illnesses associated with artificial sweeteners, the one symptom that I see most frequently is a decreased sensitivity to sugar. This is well-documented with diabetics (although it is not limited only to

Foods and Substances that Trigger Inflammation 39

diabetics), who express that sugar doesn't taste as sweet as it used to. Most people are unaware of the repercussions surrounding chemical sweeteners; it would never occur to them that these products may be having an effect on their taste buds and health.

Acquaint yourself with the following names that may appear on product labels to avoid their dangerous side effects:

- Aspartame
- Acesulfame potassium
- Alitame
- Cyclamate
- Dulcin
- Equal
- Glucin

- Kaltame
- Mogrosides
- Neotame
- Newtame
- NutraSweet
- Nutrinova
- Phenlalanine
- Saccharin

- Splenda
- Sorbitol
- Sucralose
- Twinsweet
- Sweet 'N Low
- Xylitol[13]

Top Five Worst Artificial Sweeteners

The following are the five most damaging artificial sweeteners approved for consumption in the U.S. These are all chemically manufactured molecules that do not exist in nature. Examples of products containing these sweeteners have been included.

Aspartame: NutraSweet, Equal and NatraTaste Blue
Sucralose: Splenda
Acesulfame K: Equal Spoonful, Sweet One ACE K, Sunette, and Sweet 'n Safe
Saccharin: Sweet Twin and Sweet 'N Low
Neotame: Newtame

Examples of Food, Drinks and Products that Contain Artificial Sweeteners

Be on the alert for all products and foods that contain the above chemical sweeteners. They all have a history of harmful side effects. Because these chemicals are related to many imbalances and are not recognized by the body, they would also cause inflammation.

---

13 Of these, Xylitol is the least offensive. It is being praised for reducing cavities, and as such is highly promoted by the dental community. And yet the immune system's reaction to a foreign substance entering the body has not changed, meaning that an inflammation response is still triggered by xylitol. The main complaints from ingesting xylitol have been intestinal and stomach illnesses, as well as more severe reports from pet owners.

The following are a few examples of products where artificial sweeteners are prevalent:
- Toothpaste and mouthwash
- Chewable vitamin and mineral supplements
- Cough syrup and liquid medicines (also child- and diabetic-friendly)
- Chewing gum, including nicotine gum
- Non-calorie waters and drinks (flavored fruit beverages)
- Diet fruit juices and beverages
- Soda
- Alcohol, wine and mixed drinks
- Salad dressings
- Diabetic maple syrup and jams
- Foods marketed towards diabetics
- Frozen yogurt and other frozen desserts, especially those for weight loss
- Candy (fruit based and for diabetics)
- Baked goods (breads, pastries, cookies)
- Gluten-free cereals
- Breakfast cereals
- Yogurt
- Pudding/Jell-O
- Processed snack foods
- Processed and prepared meat

These fake sweeteners are not only addictive but add to inflammation, especially if you are prone to it. Artificial sweeteners lead to all sorts of problems ranging from headaches to serious health conditions like heart disease, neurological problems, obesity, kidney disease, and much more.

Irradiated Food
Irradiation has been approved for over 50 years, and 60 countries worldwide regularly employ this food practice. One of the first foods approved for irradiation by the Food and Drug Administration (FDA) was wheat, as a means of controlling harmful insects that could enter the storage centers of grains and flours. Its use today extends into delaying ripening, preventing sprouting and mold from growing, and prolonging the shelf life of fish and meat.

Even though it is an accepted procedure, it is not without consequences. Irradiated food acts upon the body in the same way as radiation treatment. A study involving children who were fed recently irradiated wheat showed abnormal cell formation and polyploid lymph. In fact, the study was discontinued due to a surprisingly large number of abnormal cells showing up in the children's blood test samples.[14] Other studies were conducted for corroboration on rats and monkeys; the results were the same. The children and test animal's blood samples returned to normal once the wheat product was no longer consumed.

Irradiated food has shown to lower immune resistance and reduce levels of vitamins A, B complex, C, E, and K. Other problems were depressed growth rates, kidney damage, and decreased fertility.

Nitrate and Nitrites
Nitrates have been on the cancer radar for years, and are primarily found in sausages, bacon, ham, hot dogs, and cured meats. These chemicals also cause and increase inflammation. Look for products labeled additive-free, natural, and/or nitrate/nitrite free.

Trans Fats
Trans fats are found in hydrogenated oils, non-natural peanut butter, baked goods, crackers, processed and frozen food, and wraps. It is possible to eliminate these fats from your diet by reading the ingredients on the products package. Avoid foods that list hydrogenated and partially hydrogenated oil on their label.

Artificial Dyes
A petroleum and gasoline byproduct, artificial dyes are found most frequently in candy and similar items. There is a lot of controversy about the food colorings used in the United States due to many researchers linking these chemicals to disorders affecting people, from children all the way up to senior citizens. Because chemicals of this nature are associated with hormone and biological dysfunction, inflammation naturally follows. Fortunately, there are naturally-colored products sourced from carrots and beets. You can find these items and more in grocery stores and whole food stores. Look for labels that read "contains no artificial colors, flavors, or preservatives."

---

14 C. Bhaskarsmand; G. Sadasivan. Effects of Feeding Irradiated Wheat to Malnourished Children. Am J Clin Nutr. 1975, 28:2, 130-5.

Acrylamide
Acrylamide is a neurotoxin chemical, and is a result of oil being heated to extremely high temperatures. Foods like French fries, chips, and other commercial snack foods contain this inflammation-causing chemical. The National Cancer Institute has warned of the problem surrounding this cooking process for some time now. To help avoid this negative effect, lower your cooking heat and reduce cooking time. Another issue involves ordering deep fried foods at restaurants that use rancid fats, which are highly carcinogenic.

Free Radicals from Pesticides
The influence free radicals have on our body and their role in the inflammation process was covered in Chapter 3. However, since pesticides are directly related to the food we eat, it is critical that you understand that free radicals are created by the pesticide that destroys the insect. As with other damaging chemicals, pesticide-induced free radicals are accumulative.

Environmental Chemicals
Since environmental pollution is in all aspects of our daily life, it would be more appropriate to enhance your immune system through the application of herbs, supplements, and anti-inflammatory diet recommendations than to try to avoid these environmental factors. A few main sources of toxic chemicals are the exhaust fumes from motor vehicles, cigarette smoke, tap water, chemicals leached from plastic containers, modern agricultural practices and air pollution. These toxins cause inflammation in our lungs and respiratory system, among others.

Naturally, any food altering substance or process will be linked to inflammation in some way. The fact is, the food you eat shouldn't have a list of ingredients attached to it. Eat food that is free of additives that artificially enhance your food. Be sure your food selection contains a collection of vibrant colors, good fats, and quality proteins, which we'll cover in the next chapter.

CHAPTER 5

Foods That Reduce Inflammation

WHEN LOOKING TO maintain a healthy weight and optimal health, "prevention" is always a tough sell. All too often, it comes with the caveat of having to give up our favorite foods. But the truth is that not all individuals react to the same foods or substances in the same way. Something that could promote the onset of inflammation in one person might not have as pronounced an effect on another. With this in mind, the recommendations in this chapter are just that—recommendations. There is no guarantee that adding these foods to your diet will be enough to eliminate inflammation. Nor does it mean that adding in these foods will enable you to eat the foods listed in the previous chapter.

As a general guide, when looking to reduce or prevent inflammation through diet, choose foods with a lower glycemic index. If it has a label showing a list of artificial ingredients and additives, don't buy it! You should be looking to buy and cook your food from a whole, unadulterated natural or raw source.

The following food groups will naturally prevent and suppress inflammation:

Deep Water Fish: Firm white fish with scales and fins, including sardines, salmon, herring, halibut, mackerel, and trout, are among the best choices for boosting omega-3 intake.

Meat: Chicken, turkey, lamb and wild game head the list for inducing a lower inflammatory response when compared to other animal proteins.

Dairy and Milk Substitutes: The following milk substitutes are favorable when inflammation is a problem: almond milk, cashew milk, rice milk, oat milk, and coconut milk are suitable for dairy intolerant diets and far easier to digest compared to cow's milk. Make sure to avoid soy milk and soy products.

Low Glycemic Index (GI) Foods: Foods possessing a naturally lower glycemic index fall into the low-carbohydrate category. Ideally, when viewing a glycemic index chart, you are looking for foods ranging lower than 60. This means the body takes longer to break down these foods into blood glucose, especially when compared to white flour and refined sugar products. For this reason, food groups such as nuts, seeds, poultry, fish and meat have a far lower impact on blood sugar levels.

Below are examples of foods that range lowest among popular food choices, starting with the lowest selection in each category:

Fruit (Range 22–44 GI): Cherries, prunes (pitted), apple, pear, plum, peach, and orange. Dates are the highest, at 103 GI.

Vegetables (Range 20 GI): Asparagus, arugula, avocado, all sprouts, bell pepper, broccoli, Brussels sprouts, cabbage, cauliflower, celery, chard, cucumber, green beans, eggplant, mushrooms, kale, lettuce, rhubarb, spinach, scallions, zucchini, and tomatoes. Parsnips (97 GI) and baked potatoes (98 GI) range the highest.

Grains (Range 19–48 GI): 1 tablespoon rice bran (19), ½ cup pearl barely (25), 1 cup cooked oatmeal (42) and ¾ cup cooked bulgur (48). Most grains (including rice) rank high on the Glycemic Index.

Grains (Gluten-Free): For anyone who has trouble digesting gluten, inflammation will be a constant companion. The following are great and easily obtained choices that lower inflammation while aiding the waistline: brown rice, wild rice, oats, quinoa, millet, teff, amaranth, and buckwheat.

Beans/Legumes (Range 22–42 GI): Peas, whole, dried, ½ cup (22); kidney beans, ½ cup (27); lentils, ½ cup (28); lima beans (32); peas, split, yellow (32); chick peas (36); black eyed peas, ½ cup (42). Soy beans are the lowest at 14 GI per ½ cup, but soy is a known contributor to inflammation and should be avoided.

Fruit: Most fresh fruits, including apples, pineapple, papayas, cherries, blueberries, pomegranate, raspberries, and strawberries have shown not to add to the inflammation process.

Vegetables: Fresh, never canned or creamed; sweet potatoes, leafy greens, kale, spinach, and celery favor an anti-inflammatory diet.

Nuts and Seeds: Walnuts, pine nuts, almonds, sesame seeds, chia seeds, flax seeds, hemp seeds, and others are all recommended.

Legumes: All legumes, with the exception of soy, are highly recommended for their nutritional value and their ability to bind to fat molecules when eaten with a meal containing fat. While being a protein, they help to slow the absorption of sugar and carbohydrates when eaten in close proximity to these foods.

Sea Vegetables: The high mineral and trace mineral content contained in sea vegetables such as kelp, seaweed, nori, and wakame makes them a dietary must-have in squashing inflammation. These minerals boost the immune system and help support endocrine function. For convenience, sea vegetables and their properties are available in supplement form.

Maca Root: An Inflammation Superfood

Nutrient dense and antioxidant packed, many experts have put Maca root into the superfood category. Maca root is a vegetable belonging to the Brassica (cruciferous) family which grows in the high regions of the Andes Mountains in Peru. Maca is a true adaptogenic, helping the body to adapt and support the endocrine system, nervous system, and immune system, all of which are involved in the body's inflammation response.

One of the ways Maca helps to regulate inflammation is through its influence on our master regulators for stress, the pituitary gland and the hypothalamus, which helps balance out adrenal gland secretions and regulate inflammatory hormones.

Another anti-inflammatory benefit is Maca's high concentration of antioxidants, vitamins and minerals. Coupled with its balance of alkaloid and polysaccharide compounds, Maca is known for its high levels of B vitamins (riboflavin B6 and niacin B3) and vitamin C content.

Maca's minerals range from major ones like calcium and potassium to micro-nutrients which are required to manufacture hormones and enzymes in the body. All of these nutrients add up to increased energy levels and stamina, mental clarity, and the ability to better handle stress.

Maca can be purchased as a concentrated powder that may be added to liquids or smoothies.

Sugar Alternatives: Raw honey, maple syrup, stevia, agave, blackstrap molasses, and brown rice syrup top the list. For a low-glycemic choice that isn't artificial, Stevia has no affect on blood sugar and is void of calories. Raw honey is acceptable when used in moderation (½ tablespoon = 58 GI).

Healthy Oils: Cold pressed oils, including flaxseed, hemp, coconut, avocado, walnut, pumpkin, almond, and extra virgin olive oil, are all good choices. Read more about healthy oils in Chapter 3.

Spices: Research supports the ability of everyday spices to significantly dampen an inflammatory response. Four spices that show exceptional results in suppressing the immune system's inflammatory response are cloves, ginger, rosemary, and turmeric. Results can be seen even in the small, normal amounts used in everyday cooking.

Other spices that rank high as potent anti-inflammatories are curry, sage, marjoram, thyme, allspice, basil, onions, garlic, cinnamon, and cayenne. Make a point to use these whenever possible, preferably on a daily basis.

Teas to Help Reduce Inflammation

Certain plants are extremely high in beneficial properties, and when brewed or steeped into a tea, are able to treat an array of conditions. A few suggestions follow, but there are numerous choices of medicinal plants that could be incorporated into your diet to help alleviate stress, fight infection, and provide immune support to ward off inflammation.

Matcha Tea
Matcha tea is amazingly high in antioxidants, far more so than wild blueberries and chocolate (17 times the antioxidant content of wild blueberries and 7 times that of chocolate). It is best when it comes in the form of stone-ground, unfermented powder. Matcha is the most nutrient-rich green tea available.

Tulsi Tea
Tulsi Tea (also called Holy Basil) is another tea with significant levels of anti-inflammatory antioxidants that reduce the painful and dangerous inflammation associated with various forms of arthritis, cancer, and degenerative neurological disorders. Like other highly prized medicinal plants, Tulsi supports and strengthens many prominent areas of the body, such as

modulating the immune system, providing lung and bronchial support, and offering heart and vascular protection, as well as significant antioxidant and free radical scavenging abilities.

Sage Tea
Sage should be brought out of the cupboard more than those few times a year during holiday dinners. The herb sage has powerful anti-inflammatory constituents (carnosic acid and carnosol) that also contribute to its flavor. Sage is highly regarded for its antibacterial and antifungal properties. For example, using sage tea as a gargle mixed with echinacea or goldenseal tincture a few times a day can help treat and relieve strep throat. Even neurological disorders, such as Alzheimer's disease, have been researched for sage's protective anti-inflammatory benefits.

Kombucha Tea
Kombucha tea is a fermented beverage that has gained popularity recently as a potent detoxifier and for its anti-microbial and anti-cancer properties. Often referred to as the "elixir of life," Kombucha is loaded with enzymes and is a wonderful source of amino acids, antioxidants, polyphenols, probiotics, vitamins, and minerals. Kombucha also contains many vitamins (especially B12) and enzymes required by our bodies to maintain a healthy immune system.

The anti-inflammatory components of Kombucha tea are easy to assess when viewing its many system supportive properties. Kombucha is a fermented product containing probiotics (beneficial bacteria) that fights the overgrowth of harmful pathogens, including yeast and fungus, which promote inflammation.

One of Kombucha's main anti-inflammatory benefits is its rich source of glucosamines, which naturally reduce pain and inflammation, especially arthritic conditions and migraines. Glucosamines also relieve pain by increasing the production of synovial hyaluronic acid, which acts similar to NSAIDs.

Kombucha provides the body with a powerful detox, so potent that those who are newcomers to drinking Kombucha tea should take it slow. Start with 1–2 tablespoons a day to ensure your body can adjust to it. You can purchase Kombucha in bottles, but it is much cheaper to make your own.

You have now learned about how foods and plants can work to inhibit the inflammation process in the body, but there is a great deal more to maintaining your health than what has been discussed so far. The remainder of this book will focus on supporting the whole body. The body becomes ill equipped to fight disease when the main nutrients required for important tasks and functions are not being provided in the proper quantities. Starting with the next chapter, we'll be reviewing the best anti-inflammatory supplements and natural medicines to further assist in eliminating inflammation in the body.

CHAPTER 6

Assess Your Personal Health Status

A BODY THAT HAS been struggling for a long period of time, whether from malnutrition or from being burdened with bad fats and chemicals, cannot be expected to perform to the best of its ability.

This is the case for more and more people as they continue to struggle with consistently low energy levels. Without a doubt, our bodies would soar to great heights if they were to receive all the nutrients and substances (in the proper proportions) required for optimal function and restoration. The problem is, many of us come into this world with less than a fully-equipped arsenal to work with. It stands to reason that, if the mother was deficient in certain nutrients, so would be the child. For instance, many children today are being born with 50 percent lower glutathione levels than the healthy norm. This means these children have 50 percent less antioxidant protection from oxidative stress and free radical damage than a normal child. A scenario such as this can affect their young developing brains, which is just one reason why we are seeing so many behavioral imbalances. Thankfully, any missing nutrients or weak links can be made stronger by supplementing the deficient element to restore balance within the body.

Does Your Body Need to Be Propped Up?

A few simple indicators can demonstrate when a body is not nutritionally sound and functioning less than optimally. Consider the following as you evaluate the state of your body:

1. Do you feel tired most of the time?
2. Do normal activities that should be enjoyable seem to require too much effort?
3. Do you find yourself crashing, or feel you have very little stamina to complete a task or stay up past 10 pm?
4. Are you sleeping more than 8 hours and still feel tired when you wake up?
5. Do you feel depressed or overwhelmed, or have mood swings?
6. Is your memory starting to be noticeably less than it once was?
7. Has your outlook on life changed? Have you become more pessimistic or more impatient?
8. Are you experiencing skin problems like hives, dermatitis, or eczema?
9. Have imbalances with blood pressure, cholesterol levels, and higher than normal sugar (glucose) readings become part of your health status?

Many of the symptoms mentioned above indicate a lower-functioning endocrine system, which also ties into hormones, dopamine, and the neurotransmitters that induce better moods and energy. In these cases, supplementing with extra nutrients may be required to ensure all the essential needs are being met which are not being provided by the daily diet. For instance, it is very difficult to take in enough long chained fatty acids found in fish oil, especially since most people do not eat sardines and other fatty fish on a daily basis. Therefore, supplementing with cod liver oil or wild salmon oil is paramount for the body as a whole to fight off inflammation, and is necessary for proper body function and disease prevention.

Minerals are another common nutrient shortage. Trace minerals may be even harder to find in sufficient amounts in today's agricultural procedures. The two main minerals in the body that have the most jobs to perform are magnesium and zinc. These two minerals perform many more tasks compared to other nutrients in the body (with the exception of essential fatty acids), and yet our bodies are chronically in deficit for these crucial minerals. Conditions that can result from nutrient deficits include anemia and other illnesses of general weakness. Thankfully, such problems are *not* insurmountable. Once a weakness is known, a proper nutritional solution can be instituted to help prop up any weak links and support any system imbalance.

Examples of Conditions Related to a Nutrient Deficiency

To discuss each of the numerous illnesses and complaints related to specific vitamins, minerals would be a book in and of itself, so we have restricted our discussion here to a few examples that illustrate how something that may seem insignificant can actually have a great impact on how your body performs.

One example, previously discussed in Chapter 1, demonstrates that inherited enzyme weakness leading to eczema can be remedied by the alpha-gamma linolenic acids found in evening primrose oil. Another involves inflammatory bowel disorders like Crohns' disease, which can be addressed through the application of magnesium. The carrier protein for this mineral is often impaired and must be supported for the body to have any success at proper functioning and healing.

Neurological disorders, on the other hand, may be due to a lack of a particular amino acid (as seen in cases of autism, along with low levels of glutathione and protein absorption problems). Deficient amounts of certain B vitamins may be a major contributor to schizophrenia. A build-up of fungus reaching the brains of people who suffer with bipolar disorder may occur due to a lack of beneficial gut bacteria. (Without a proper balance of good flora, our immune system is greatly compromised; 20 percent of the thyroid gland's functions depend on our body's good bacteria.)

The following nutritional suggestions are ones I routinely find to be either missing or insufficiently supplied by people's diet. There are always individual needs—either determined by inherent weakness, poor quality nutrition, or specific demands brought about by certain illnesses—but the suggestions below are general purpose, and designed to help pick up energy levels, boost immunity, enhance circulation and promote better moods.

- Iodine: Required for thyroid function and production of Thyroid Stimulation Hormone (TSH). Required daily.
- Trace minerals: Algae (blue or green) and seaweed contain many trace minerals that land plants do not possess.
- Magnesium and zinc: Work together to promote immune function, among many other tasks

- L-Tyrosine: An amino acid and the main energy component in the body. Most people over the age of 19 are deficient in this all-important amino acid.
- Omega-3 fatty acids: Incredibly important; involved in every system, function and all other components of the body.
- Vitamin E: A main antioxidant in the body. Aids circulation.
- Vitamin D3: Obtained through exposure to sunlight. Those in areas of low light may require supplementation.
- B vitamins: B vitamins like to be in balance with each other, although individual vitamins are needed for specific conditions.
- Probiotics (Lacto-bacillus and acidophilus): A major component of our immune system.
- Chlorophyll: Helpful when there is a lack of live food and fresh greens. It is similar to our own blood matrix, providing cleansing and remineralization.
- Live enzymes and antioxidants: Found abundantly in live food that has not been cooked (salads, fresh juice, raw fruits and vegetables).

Assess Your Level of Nutrition

It is in everyone's best interest to provide their body with as many necessary nutrients as possible. But does your level of nutrition measure up? Do a mental assessment of what you eat on a daily basis. Have you introduced any extra supplementation to help pick up what you routinely do not eat enough of?

A few of the following points may help you evaluate your level of daily nutrition:

1. Is most or all of the food you eat cooked?
2. How much of your intake is processed or pre-packaged?
3. How often do you eat fast food or junk food?
4. Does your daily food intake consist mainly of starch and protein sources?
5. Do you regularly consume diet soda, energy drinks and other sugary liquids?
6. Do you smoke cigarettes or drink alcohol on a regular basis?

7. Do you rarely cook and eat out often?
8. Is your diet high in sugar (baked goods, pastries, cookies and candy)?
9. Is your consumption of fruits and vegetables low in comparison to all other food?

If several of the above suggestions are a main part of your diet, inflammation throughout the body is also likely to be part of your daily existence. Feeling sluggish and tired would also be expected.

The point of this exercise is to see if your diet is adequate in its level of vitamins, minerals, antioxidants, enzymes, and essential fatty acids. We all need live food; we need the antioxidants and enzymes found in fruits and vegetables, as well as the vitamins and minerals, to ensure certain essential elements are being met. Extra nutritional supplements may also be required for any items that are not routinely covered in normal intake, like fish oil and iodine.

For a guide to eating more optimally, read through the anti-inflammatory diet protocols in Chapter 10. This diet plan is not just for reducing inflammation, but presents a way to eat that best suits our nutritional and biochemical needs.

The next chapter will continue to assist you in evaluating your nutritional requirements while quelling inflammation. In addition to learning about specific nutrients that are highly beneficial for reducing and warding off inflammation, you will learn about how these elements work in the body, which can then help you boost your weaker and lower-functioning areas.

CHAPTER 7

Natural Supplementation for Reversing Inflammation

A WELL-ROUNDED ANTI-INFLAMMATORY PROTOCOL, such as the one outlined in this chapter, will include foods that reduce inflammation, antioxidants, live enzymes, and anti-inflammatory supplements. The additional benefit of extra supplementation is in providing higher amounts of isolated nutrients that have been proven to control and affect inflammation all the while offering protection.

That said, while natural anti-inflammatories are uniquely powerful remedies, they need to be paired with healthful lifestyle choices that work to deactivate all the major stimulants to chronic inflammation in order to reach their full effectiveness. Supplements will not replace poor eating habits. The reversal process for healing and restoration significantly slows down when several vitamins and minerals are in very short supply, especially those required by the immune system and for performing body functions. One way to boost this process is through juicing raw greens, vegetables and fruits, to obtain their enzymes, antioxidants and concentrated nutrients, to offset a less-than-optimal diet.

In this chapter, we'll examine the wide variety of natural anti-inflammatories available, their numerous applications, and how to achieve best results consistently. As we'll be discussing the importance of avoiding nutrient deficiencies throughout this chapter, it may be helpful to define some of the terms we use to describe these essential elements.

Minerals

Minerals are inorganic substances drawn from plants and animals and which serve our body as essential chemical building blocks. Minerals are critical for creating certain key enzymes that enhance or initiate the chemical reactions necessary for life itself.

Minerals are a vital and mandatory component for all cellular reactions throughout the body. A process known as mineral chelation occurs in the intestinal tract, in which dissolved minerals convert into mineral salts and then become ions (a molecule with one or more electrons added or absent which possesses either a negative or a positive charge). The chelation process provides stability, allowing these ions to pass through the gut wall and into the bloodstream more easily.

The main composition of minerals within the body is this chelated form. To ensure a successful chelation process, minerals should be taken with a protein. To aid this process, the amino acids found in protein (along with stomach enzymes and acids) are all required to be present in adequate amounts. In this way, mineral ions are successfully directed to their destinations, such as our bones, organs and glands.

Vitamins

Vitamins are organic substances which the body depends on to catalyze certain reactions.

Vitamins work either alone or as cofactors with other chemical elements or enzymes. When the term *essential* is applied to specific vitamins and minerals, it indicates that a deficiency of anyone of these elements could lead to an impaired function, causing symptoms of stress and disease or ultimately even death. There is an intricate dance taking place throughout our body every day, which requires a proper balance of nutrients in order to support a healthy, functioning body.

Vitamins fall into two categories: water soluble and fat soluble. The main difference between them is water soluble vitamins (like vitamin C and B) dissolve in water before the body can absorb them, whereas fat soluble vitamins (vitamins A, D, E and K) dissolve in fat and can be stored in the body. Water soluble vitamins must therefore be taken in daily, and are found in plants and animals and often taken in supplement form. They are excreted in the urine when taken in larger amounts; therefore, at those times when you may require higher dosages of vitamins (such as vitamin

C, for fighting an infection), the suggestion would be to take smaller dosages spread throughout the day rather than a megadose all at once. Fat soluble vitamins, which require a fat molecule for transportation throughout the body, are absorbed through the small intestine (via dietary fat) and excreted slowly from the body. When there is an excess of these nutrients, they will be stored in the body's fatty tissue and liver.

Vitamin C
Vitamin C is impressive on many levels. A powerful antioxidant, vitamin C is highly endorsed for combating cancer and inflammation. Vitamin C is required for the repair of connective tissue, as well as the production of collagen. If you are undergoing intense exercise or recovering from an infection or injury, consider temporarily taking a higher dosage of vitamin C, 1–2 g daily.

Suggested dosage for optimum health: 2000–4000 mg, divided throughout the day.

Good food sources: Citrus fruit, strawberries, kiwi, bell peppers, berries, cantaloupe, mango and a variety of vegetables.

Vitamin A
To enhance healing due to injury or from too much strenuous exercise, the recommended dosage of vitamin A would be 10,000 IU daily for 1–2 weeks derived from fish oils. A few areas requiring vitamin A support include your immune system, vision, reproductive systems, bone growth, tooth development and proper functioning of our heart, lungs and kidneys.

Vitamin D (Fat Soluble)
When the body becomes deficient in vitamin D, it is virtually impossible for proper absorption of calcium. Fat soluble vitamin D can be found naturally in fish oil, and is best absorbed with a meal that contains some form of fat—preferably a good fat source. Milk is another source of fat soluble vitamin D, as long as most of the fat has not been removed. But if you have challenges in getting enough vitamin D, sunshine is still the most reliable source.

Good sources for fat soluble vitamin D can be found in the following foods.

- Fish liver oils (wild salmon and cod liver oils), fatty fish (salmon, mackerel, halibut, sardines, and herring
- Egg yolks
- Fortified milk, orange juice and cereals
- Dried shiitake mushrooms

Vitamin D (Water Soluble)
For the most potent form of vitamin D, choose vitamin D3 (cholecalciferol), the active form of vitamin D. Do not purchase vitamin D2, as it is not as biologically active or as safe as vitamin D3. The recommended dosage for vitamin D3, as put forward by the Vitamin D council, is a minimum of 1000 IU per 25 pounds of body weight.

Vitamin E
Vitamin E is stored in the body's fatty tissue and is perhaps best known for its highly motivated assault on free radicals. Vitamin E also prevents the blood from clotting and boosts the immune system. Always choose natural sourced vitamin E because it is 50 times more powerful than the synthetic from.

Now, to debunk a popular misconception: several years ago, a severely flawed vitamin E study using synthetic vitamin E stated that a moderate to high dosage of vitamin E may increase a person's risk for heart attack. The results of this study were held for three years, to benefit the release of a heart medication. Unfortunately, once the facts of this study were exposed, it was never publicly recanted.

Suggested dosage: 400 IU per day or 800–1200 IU divided up through the day for extreme hot flashes and circulation problems.

Good sources of Vitamin E can be found in wheat germ, nuts, seeds (almonds, sunflower seeds, sesame, walnuts and hazelnuts).

Vitamin K2 (MK-7)
There are two basic types of Vitamin K: K1 and K2. The different forms of vitamin K carry out specific duties in the body. Vitamin K1 is found in green plants, especially their juice (chlorophyll), and maintains healthy blood clotting in the body; whereas K2 is produced by bacteria in our gut.

A study released at the International Nutrition and Diagnostics Conference in the Czech Republic announced the value of K2 (MK-7) for the prevention of inflammation. The study demonstrated that K2 (MK-7) prevents inflammation by blocking pro-inflammatory markers (monocytes) produced by white blood cells.

K2 isn't as widely available in our food as K1; the Japanese food natto is by far the richest source of K2 (although some types of cheese contain K2, with Gouda ranking the highest). If you feel your diet is insufficient, pick it up with 150 mcg; there is no evidence of overdosing occurring, even with very high amounts of this vitamin.

Essential Fatty Acids (EFAs)

The word "essential" has never had more meaning. Without these fats in their proper proportion, it would not be possible to remain well—let alone pain-free—throughout one's lifetime. Huge strides have been made in science showing us the necessity for adequate amounts of EFAs for disease prevention and for fully functioning body systems. Of these, omega 3s are the ones most sought after by the body (typically found in fish and seed oils), especially since our diets have been traditionally high in the omega 6 fatty acids found in vegetable and grain cooking oils. (As stated earlier, the proper ratio for optimum balance in the body of omega 6 fatty acids compared to omega 3 fatty acids is a 1:1 ratio, whereas most people maintain a 20:1 or even 30:1 ratio).

Our body's inflammation response, immune response, tissue repair and formation of every cell membrane all require an omega 3 fatty acid. Knowing that, it isn't hard to understand why our bodies aren't able to alleviate pain or the progression of chronic inflammatory problems on their own. People with chronic inflammation taking fish oils a few times a day have significantly less pain and a better quality of life. When choosing a quality blend of fish oil, look for the ratio between DHA (docosahexaenoic acid) and EPA (eicosapentaenoic acid) to be approximately 2:1. Depending on the severity of one's complaint, the following suggested dosage of fish oil would not be uncommon: 1000–3000 mg three times a day with food.

> **Green Lipped Mussel Oil**
>
> Green lipped mussel oil is being hailed for its restorative and anti-inflammatory powers, especially in the area of joint and knee pain and forms of arthritis. Whether it be the mussels themselves or the extracted oil or powder form, the properties and benefits are highly impressive. They are quite unique compared to most whole food supplements: green lipped mussels contain omega 3 fatty acids, proteins, minerals, vitamins, glycoproteins, healthy enzymes, chondroitin sulphate, glycosaminoglycans, polysaccharides and polypeptides.
>
> Because of its unusual collection of nutrients, this supplement has been an effective treatment for joint health, preservation of mobility, rebuilding cartilage, skin problems, heart health and those suffering with chronic pain, fibromyalgia, rheumatoid arthritis, osteoarthritis, lupus and other respiratory illnesses such as asthma and chronic bronchitis.
>
> Improvements were noted in study results using 200–350 mg of oil per day.

Gut Flora

Our body's individual microbiome environment—the community of microorganisms that perform a number of crucial functions in our body—is our constant companion and caregiver throughout our life, without which we could not survive. And, because these beneficial bacteria are key to a well-functioning immune system, it's only natural that they help ward off chronic inflammation. We have 100,000 billion viable microbes in our intestines; of the fecal mass excreted from the body, 85 percent is biomass (bacteria).

The biggest threat to these 200 different species (7000 strains) is antibiotics. Considering the prominent place these microbes hold in our body, it isn't hard to see how chronic inflammatory intestinal diseases like Crohn's and colitis can besiege the body as a result of our gut's having been napalmed by antibiotics. To support this crucial system, supplement daily with probiotics and eat fermented foods like kefir, natto and sauerkraut.

Antioxidants

In nature, antioxidants are the pigments in plants that give them their intense and brilliant colors. But more importantly, antioxidants are a major part of our body's defense team, and come in many different categories. Even though mankind has been consuming these nutrients for thousands of years, only recently have comprehensive studies taken place to understand the complex role they play. By incorporating foods rich in antioxidant qualities, dangerous free radicals will be neutralized, preventing degenerative diseases, while also providing protection against infections and repairing damaged genes.

Antioxidants are classified into two groups: water soluble (hydrophilic) or lipids (hydrophobic). They are also grouped by their response time in the body, as fast acting and slow acting. A slow acting antioxidant example is classified as a complex organic antioxidant (such as phenolics) while a fast acting antioxidant would be something closer to vitamin C.

The following are an assortment of potent antioxidants and their sources, which can help to support your immune system and manage chronic inflammation.

Alpha Lipoic Acid
Referred to as a semi-essential nutrient, alpha lipoic acid is a key player in the antioxidant recycling process and therefore is of value when found in multiple supplement formulas. It is the only nutrient that is both water and fat soluble.

For maximum benefit, it is suggested that persons take higher dosages, ranging from 100–900 mg per day.

Beta-Carotene (and Other Carotenoids)
Antioxidants such as beta-carotene and other carotenoids have been agreed upon by many scientists (including those at Yale University School of Medicine) as the antioxidant best suited to protect us against chronic illnesses. Plants are protected by their antioxidant compounds, and the people who consume these properties are similarly protected.

Beta-carotene and alpha-carotene are water soluble vitamins found in yellow and orange fruits and vegetables, but as these can merge with other phyto-nutrients, they may also be found in red and pink foods. Alpha-carotene is classified as pro-vitamin A, which means it can be converted into the active form of vitamin A known as retinol. Similarly, beta-carotene can also be converted into vitamin A. Thanks to their positive effect neutralizing free radicals in the body, clinical evidence and research studies supports the addition of carotenoids to help prevent abnormal cellular growth and activity involved in aliments such as cancer, cardiovascular health, vision, memory, dementia and diabetes.

Food sources include: carrots, squash, pumpkin, peppers, tomatoes, oranges, lemons, mangos, papaya and sweet potatoes. Certain green vegetables also have high amounts of carotenoids, such as kale, spinach, collard greens, thyme and cilantro.

Astaxanthin
Found in many aquatic species, astaxanthin is a red carotenoid (fat-soluble) which is gaining notoriety for its enhanced ability to protect the nervous system, brain and eyes.

Astaxanthin is also gaining popularity due to the unique characteristic that, when recycling free radical electrons, astaxanthin does not become ineffective after eliminating these extra electrons, like other antioxidants. It then follows that astaxanthin is one of the most powerful carotenoids in the unique way it protects plants, animals and sea life.

Astaxanthin protects the body from cellular damage associated with high oxidative foods and reduces inflammation in body tissues and joints. Being fat soluble, coupling astaxanthin with fish oil has been shown to work effectively.

Suggested dosage: 4–12 mg per day. Good sources include Nordic Naturals, Carlson Labs and Natural Factors.

Falcarinol
Falcarinol is a natural pesticide and plant antioxidant which imparts its same benefits to people who consume the foods it's contained in. Carrots are especially high in this protective nutrient, which shows ten times the ability to inhibit cancer cells compared to beta-carotene. Juice or cook carrots whole to retain this element.

Lycopene
Lycopene is one of the most respected members of the carotenoid family—and also one of the most beneficial. Lycopene possesses the capability to eliminate singlet oxygen radicals, one of the most damaging of all free radicals. Oxygen singlet radicals are highly reactive byproducts of oxidation, formed during the metabolism of polyunsaturated fatty acids and has shown to be extremely damaging to healthy cells.

Red in color, lycopene is found in such foods as tomatoes, pink grapefruit, watermelon and papaya.

Resveratrol
The polyphenolic phytochemical resveratrol, found in grapes and berries, has earned a reputation as a potent protective agent against inflammatory cytokines and free radicals. These protective chemicals also elevate glutathione in the body and further the formation of antioxidant enzymes.

Sulphur Phyto-Nutrients
Sulphorane, indoles, isothiocyanates, and alpha lipoic acid (mentioned earlier) are all sulphur phyto-nutrients found in such vegetables as asparagus, broccoli, cauliflower, mustard greens and onions. Studies show that sulforaphane stimulates antioxidant enzymes NFE2L2 or Nrf-2 (nuclear factor erythroid-derived 2), which regulates the expression of protective antioxidant proteins against oxidative damage brought on by inflammation and injury. Phytochemicals (like glucosinolates) found in cruciferous vegetables are enzymatically converted into sulforaphane and other chemical constituents, which research has revealed to work at a much deeper level of the body. These compounds actually influence our genes to increase the production of alkaline defense mechanisms involved in the detoxification process.

Bromelain
An enzyme sourced from pineapple, bromelain has been shown to be especially useful in assisting healing from most physical injuries and improve absorption of other nutrients. It most often accompanies digestive aid formulas and proteolytic systemic enzyme formulas, and goes well coupled with certain herbs like turmeric to enhance absorbability.

Epigallocatechin-3-gallate (EGCG)
EGCG is a type of catechin, which is most abundantly found in green tea (7380 mg per 100 grams), white tea (4245 mg per 100 grams), and (in smaller amounts) in black tea. For the most part, these catechins are converted to thearubigins and theaflavins. Smaller amounts can be found in plums, apple skin, pecans, hazelnuts and carob.

A-Adenosyl Methionine (SAMe)
A major application for SAMe is in pain management, as it helps us to deal with pain in a rational manner. This is because the mechanisms that make it possible for us to deal with pain and inflammation are regulated by one of the peptides (serotonin) that SAMe produces. SAMe is created within the body when the amino acid methionine joins up with energy-producing adenosine triphosphate (ATP), providing the fuel for our body's systems, cartilage and joint material, as well as organs (in particular, the brain and liver).

However, this barely scratches the surface of the benefits and therapeutic uses of SAMe. Even as you are reading this, your body is doing everything it possibly can to manufacture SAMe, since it is the element that is essential for the billions of chemical reactions that take place in our cells on a continual basis. Since its discovery, SAMe has swept Europe, becoming one of most prescribed remedies (even topping the sales of Prozac). In the U.S., millions of people take this supplement on a regular basis for everything from pain to age-related memory problems like Alzheimer's.

SAMe supports all manner of pain and inflammation relief, and helps with the associated symptoms of fatigue and depression. For arthritic pain, take 600 mg 2–3 times a day. If you are also taking anti-depressants, take 800 mg 2–3 times a day.

Proteolytic Enzymes

Proteolytic enzymes (or proteases) refer to the various enzymes that break down protein in the body. For these enzymes to work effectively, they must get past the body's harsh stomach acid in order to reach the small intestine, where it can be absorbed into the bloodstream. To enable this process, supplements containing these enzymes have an enteric coating to allow for maximum protection. Health care professionals recommend these powerful enzymes because of their ability to dissolve fibrin, detoxify the body, break up mineral compounds and cleanse the blood.

Serrapeptase and Proteinase
Serrapeptase and proteinase are two naturally occurring enzymes that have demonstrated significant anti-inflammatory properties. Serrapeptase is derived from silkworms, and is showing to be one of the most potent and effective anti-inflammatory (protein-eating) enzymes. These enzymes and a few others are widely used for their ability to rid the body of excess fibrin. For this reason they have huge applications in the fight against cancer and breaking up scar tissue, plus the removal of fibrinogen (which thickens the blood like ketchup, promoting stroke or aneurysm).

Nattokinase Enzyme
Another fibrin-dissolving enzyme, nattokinase is often used for cardiovascular complications to free up circulation.

Superoxide Dismutase (SOD) Enzyme
Superoxide sismutase is a potent antioxidant regarded for its ability to break down potentially harmful oxygen molecules in cells, thereby preventing tissue damage. Among its many profound benefits is excellent inflammation control.

Other proteolytic enzymes that assist the digestive process in breaking down proteins include pancreatin, bromelain, papain, trypsin, chymotrypsin and peptidase.

CHAPTER 8

Purchasing Herbal and Supplement Products

Choosing a Quality Herbal Product

One of my earliest lessons in phytochemistry was learning the journey a medicinal plant takes on its way to becoming a dietary supplement. The main concern then, as it is now, is regarding the amount of active ingredients the plant is able to retain—even before it reaches the processing stage. Imagine a large load of plant material leaving Europe, destined for the United States. Government regulations require that these plants be sprayed with fungicides and pesticides before taking their journey across the ocean. Having landed in New York, the plants are then stored in a warehouse where they are once again sprayed, as a precaution against dangerous foreign material entering the country. In some cases, this cargo can remain in its holding container for up to a year. I ask the same question I was posed as a student: "What medicinal properties do you think are still retained in these plant parts?"

I am not suggesting that this is the norm for all products coming into this country. But I do advocate for making sure that the products you purchase come from a trustworthy, quality source. Consider checking the products you are considering with Brunswick Labs and other reputable websites which list product brands that have gone through rigorous testing for their ingredients and for any contamination. Remember, if it seems too good to be true (or is very inexpensive), it probably is. For this reason, it's best to watch out for online or mail order brands and catalogues. Herbal products that are labeled "standardized" or "wild crafted" often implies that you will be getting the amount of plant product that should be in the container, and not have any replaced with other plants and fillers. You also have a much better chance that the plants medicinal properties are still intact and not dissipated or laden with chemicals.

It is important to note that more than 30 percent of herbal products do not measure up to quality criteria. You also do not need to purchase the most expensive product in order for the product to work. There are mid-ranged and reasonably priced products available. Sometimes, a knowledgeable person who works in the store you are purchasing from can offer guidance. Otherwise, check before you buy.

For a few suggestions of trustworthy brands, try:

- Seroyal
- Genestra
- Ultra Laboratories
- Natural Factors
- General Nutrition
- Nature's Bounty
- Natrol
- Sundown
- Sangisters

How to Choose a Quality Supplement

It is always wonderful to have choices in our lives, yet when these choices become overwhelming or confusing, the end result is often doing nothing at all. The U.S. dietary supplement industry is estimated at $27 billion, which implies a vast amount of products to choose from. The following tips will assist in choosing a product that lives up to its label.

Look for Tested Formulas
Look to see if the product's ingredients or the formula's benefit have gone through clinical trials and has supportive data. If at all possible, try to choose products that have been put through human clinical trials. It isn't that animal studies are invalid, but I have often come across inappropriate dosages being given to test animals that would never be given to a human—the dosage would be astronomically high if the same study structure was carried out in human trials. I find this to be more prevalent for plants and their extracts; what's worse, most times there aren't any clinical human trials to reference.

For additional help, there are websites whose focus is product safety and control, such as Consumer Lab (www.consumerlab.com), which focuses on vitamin, mineral and nutrient supplements, and Brunswick Lab (www.

brunswicklabs.com) when choosing an herbal product. The Natural Products Association (www.npainfo.org) can also be a big help.

Look for Quality Ingredients

A reputable supplement manufacturer will formulate their products based on scientific research. Look for verification of quality for ingredients by visiting their websites. If you are still not satisfied, call the company and inquire about quality control measures. Look into the route used for product testing and processing; this can be very important, especially depending on whether it is second and third party.

Testing should match manufacturer claims for product strength, purity and ingredient integrity of the properties being used, singularly or in a formulation. Find out what country the ingredients are sourced from, since raw material from certain counties does not meet the "standardized" criteria. Remember that brochures and labels are not always accurate in their claims!

Look for Chemical Additives
When looking to purchase natural supplements, you'll want to avoid products with an abundance of unnecessary chemical additives. Magnesium stearate, for example, is the main compound used in the manufacturing of vitamin supplements and medications, and is formed by adding a magnesium ion to stearic acid. Its presence allows for more efficient production and greater yields, and adds a lubricating quality to the machinery, yet recent research has revealed that stearic acid suppresses the T cells in our immune system (natural killer cells) and affects the structural integrity of our cell membranes, causing a collapse which can ultimately destroy cell function.

Read product labels carefully; companies are required to disclose additional processing agents. In addition, look for company standards for quality assurance, including ISO 9001, ISO 17025 and Good Manufacturing Processes (GMP) certifications.

Choose products that avoid ingredients that may cause food intolerance or sensitivity, as well as harmful chemicals. Be on the watch for the following items:
- Artificial colors
- Artificial flavors
- Phthalates
- Magnesium stearate
- Talc
- Titanium dioxide

- Fish
- Dairy
- Wheat
- Yeast
- Gluten
- GMOs

Look for Source Absorbability Factor
Read the Supplement Facts panel on the product for more detailed information on each ingredient's source. This is an area that can show how absorbable the ingredients may be. For example, when an ingredient listing is followed by "co-enzymated," it indicates a higher absorption rate, while the term "chelation" (associated with mineral supplements) is a method used to improve bioavailability of minerals. Additional names associated with chelated minerals include magnesium succinate, calcium citrate and others.

For those with have assimilation challenges due to low hydrochloric acid, a collection of different mineral sources in a product can be helpful. For instance, sources of calcium may include carbonate, ascorbate, malate, and citrate as available sources.

How to Make Tea Using Plant Parts

When making tea from natural herbs and plant parts, it's important to tailor your method of brewing to the material you'll be preparing. For example, the aerial parts of a plant—such as the flowers and leaves—would call for an infusion process, whereas the hard woody parts and roots of plants will require a decoction process.

Infusion: The process most people think of when they imagine making tea, infusion involves putting 1 teaspoon of dried herb in a cup and filling with boiling water. Let it steep for 10–15 minutes and consume. For fresh herbs, try 1 tablespoon of herb per cup of boiling water.

Decoction: In order to draw out the medicinal properties from the hard, dense parts of plants, they must go through a tincture or decoction process. To make decoction tea, measure 1 teaspoon dried herb per cup of water in a stainless steel pot and bring to a boil. Once boiled, lower to a simmer for an additional 12–15 minutes.

Now that you know how to purchase a quality product, you will have more success at choosing a high-quality, naturally sourced remedy to alleviate your pain and discomfort. The next chapter is loaded with great suggestions for restoring comfort in your daily life while also increasing general mobility.

CHAPTER 9

Reversing Inflammation —Naturally

EVEN THE MOST troublesome inflammatory conditions that afflict mankind can be treated—and *are* being treated worldwide—with herbal medicine. How many times has it been said, "Nature holds the cure?" The fact is that our biological needs can be met by our evolutionary environment. The plant kingdom is abundant with anti-inflammatory specimens, many of which are currently being used in the production of steroidal anti-inflammatory medications.

Sadly, for a natural substance to become a pharmacological agent, it must become a synthetic compound so it can be patented. Natural substances cannot be patented; as a result, our most frequently-used remedies no longer have the ability to grow tissue and can no longer interrelate with the hundred thousand protein molecules in our body. One of the most appreciated attributes of these patented drugs is their ability to block pain and sensory communication rapidly throughout the body. Unfortunately, this benefit does not come without a price; as already discussed, anti-inflammatory drugs and prescription medications cannot follow the holistic pathway in the body, and are therefore unrecognizable to our immune system. Instead of boosting the anti-inflammatory pathways, they suppress them while the pro-inflammatory pathways become even more enhanced.

While a plant in its whole, unadulterated state (from which drugs are originally sourced), it cannot act as potently as medication. Like the food we eat, natural remedies take more time to integrate into our bodies, but their active ingredients are also balanced when taken into the body. For that reason, they are not life-threatening or as dangerous. For instance, a plant species that is classified as a nervine (plant source for anti-depressants) would also possess properties for healing the nerve sheath and for soothing inflammation while calming the heightened response from the glands.

It is important to remember that even though there are wonderful and plentiful natural remedies to choose from, the body works as a whole. Pay attention to dietary triggers for inflammation, as well as the quality of your nutritional intake. Do you require supplementation to address energy levels, support circulation, and boost the immune system? Are your liver and eliminative systems working properly and well enough for optimum detoxification? Look at all the health complaints you have and evaluate where improvement is needed, or else get assistance from a health care provider that understands and can address the root cause of your complaint.

Anti-Inflammatory Herbs

Natural restorative herbal remedies are beginning to see proper recognition for their place at the forefront of healthful supplements. Many of these plants and extracts show the complex and integrated ways in which an herbal remedy can work. Their valuable components continue to demonstrate new and effective applications, including anti-inflammatory, antioxidative, and anti-asthmatic properties. Some of these properties include flavonoids, alkaloids, saponins, anthraquinones, and terpenoids. These properties and more, when utilized properly, have numerous pharmacological uses.

Shosaikoto

Shosaikoto is a traditional Chinese remedy that, for over 2,000 years, has been used to treat many symptom complaints, including inflammation and liver-related problems. But now, recent clinical studies support the application of shosaikoto for the reduction of adverse effects induced by Western medicines. One of the main findings involved its positive influence on patients taking steroid drugs like prednisolone. The study was aimed at decreasing drug use while maintaining the therapeutic effect of the medication. Combination therapy with glucocorticoids or anti-tumor drugs and shosaikoto showed positive results in multiple cases: the adverse effects upon the liver from using steroids were decreased, as was the dosage, while still keeping its therapeutic effect.

Shosaikoto has also enabled patients with rheumatoid arthritis, chronic hepatitis, and nephritis to withdraw from their glucocorticoids. Shosaikoto is available for purchase through online retailers like Amazon.

Curcumin

Turmeric, the yellow pigment popularly known as the main ingredient in Asian curry cuisine, is currently being heavily researched to ascertain the positive properties of its prime component, curcumin. Curcumin has been found to possess profound anti-inflammatory properties; the one remaining issue involves curcumin's poor rate of absorption and the rate at which the body purges it from its system.

The product Theracurmin was developed to address these issues, and when tested against all other commercial brands, ranked far superior in terms of its absorption rate.[15] The reason for its success is due to its particle size (100 times smaller than the average curcumin powder particle) which radically increases its solubility in water, resulting in an unequalled absorption rate. The benefits of Theracurmin range from reduced tissue damage caused by inflammation to improved heart and liver function. In addition, quality of life improvements for cancer patients was also noted.

Boswellia

Boswellia is on the fast track to earning fame in the family of medicinal plants. It has caught the attention of many scientists because it can actually block the lethal pro-inflammatory enzyme called 5-lipoxygenase (5-LOX), the first enzyme in the metabolic pathway leading to the synthesis of leukotrienes. Until recently, attempts to inhibit this potent contributor to inflammatory conditions have proven very ineffective. Boswellia's ability to block 5-LOX is turning out to be an important element in the treatment of asthma and cancer, along with other life-threatening illnesses.

Remarkably, the anti-inflammatory compounds found in Boswellia inhibit both 5-LOX and HLE (human leukocyte elastase). Boswellic acids decrease the activity of HLE, which is another pro-inflammatory enzyme. This enzyme is associated with a long list of chronic conditions such as rheumatoid arthritis, pulmonary emphysema, chronic bronchitis, cystic fibrosis, and acute respiratory illnesses. These and more are all linked to inflammation.

When purchasing Boswellia, look for a product that contains a standardized content of 60–65 percent boswellic acid, the herb's active ingredient. Suggested dosage: 300 mg three times a day for conditions of chronic

---

15 Sasaki H, Sunagawa Y, Takahashi K, et al. Innovative preparation of Curcumin for improved oral bioavailability. Biol Pharm Bull. 2011;34(5):660-5.

pain, asthma, arthritic complaints, inflammatory bowel disease, and sports-related injuries.

Cat's Claw
Cat's claw, a woody vine native to rainforest areas in South America, has undergone many studies to demonstrate how its extracts can be potent anti-inflammatories and powerful antioxidants. Cat's claw's success at overcoming dangerous superoxide and peroxyl radicals has revealed that its potency exceeds that of many other extracts found in fruits, vegetables, and other medicinal plants.

In addition, Mark JS Miller and his colleagues conducted studies that showed Cat's claw's immense benefits for limiting cartilage degradation by suppressing catabolism and activating local IGF-1 anabolic pathways.[16] It has also shown to be an inhibitor of NF-kappaB.

Suggested dosage: Commercial preparations may vary in dosage and standardization of cat's claw active ingredients. The suggested dosage of a cat's claw preparation is up to 350 mg daily, standardized to contain 8 percent carboxy alkyl esters. Tincture: 20 drops three times per day.

Horseweed (Conyza Canadensis)
Also known as colt's-tail, fleabane, and hogweed, horseweed is a member of the Asteraceae family and a relative to many known plants in North America. Its mineral content registers very high for potassium, calcium and phosphorus. Horseweed leaves are edible, either in a salad or cooked (similar to spinach).

For many years now, research has been looking into the many benefits of horseweed, including anti-inflammatory, antifungal, and antimicrobial activities, as well as antibacterial, antioxidant, and cytotoxic activities (the ability to kill cells; chemotherapy is cytotoxic therapy).

One aspect of horseweed's highly-rated anti-inflammatory activity is owed to its eight sesquiterpenes. Sesquiterpene lactones are most often found in the leaves and flowers of plants and are valued for the following

---

[16] Miller MJ, Ahmed S, Bobrowski P, Haqqi TM. The chrondoprotective actions of a natural product are associated with the activation of IGF-1 production by human chondrocytes despite the presence of IL-1beta. BMC Complement Altern Med. 2006 Apr 7;6:13.

benefits: anti-inflammatory, antiprotozoal, antibacterial, antimicrobial, and digestive bitter.

Conzya extract has other impressive actions, two of which are anti-aggregatory (preventing the aggregation of platelets) and the prevention of peroxynitrite-related diseases like cardiovascular and inflammatory diseases. (Peroxynitrite is an oxidant and nitrating intermediary that can damage a wide range of cells, including proteins and DNA, due to its oxidizing properties).

Devil's Claw (Harpagophytum procumbens)
This plant hails from Africa, and gets its foreboding name from its claw-shaped fruit. Ever since this plant's rhizome was scientifically discovered in 1958, its strong anti-inflammatory properties have been compared to cortisone and phenylbutazone. Devil's claw has been widely used for all forms of arthritis and pain and swelling in joints. For this reason it has great applications for rheumatoid arthritis and dietary intolerances.

Devil's claw is easily purchased from stores who sell health supplements.

Suggested preparation: Tincture, 1–2 ml 3–5 times per day; decoction tea, 1 teaspoon per cup of water, and drink three times a day for at least one month, continuing as needed.

Sinomenine (Sinomenium acutum)
Sinomenine is native to Japan and China. A climbing plant, sinomenine contains a potent alkaloid found in its roots. Because this plant possesses this analgesic alkaloid, it is mainly used in the pharmaceutical field. Sinomenine's usage extends to neuralgia and rheumatic diseases, and is used traditionally as a treatment for arthritis and rheumatism. Sinomenine's strong anti-inflammatory effect is achieved through its powerful histamine release. In addition to several other health promoting benefits, sinomenine has shown to be effective for lowering blood pressure and as an antitussive (to suppress a cough).

In clinical trials, sinomenine inhibited inflammatory cytokine production and degranulation of mass cells in connective tissue (joint and skin).

Dosage suggestion: High dosages of sinomenine can be toxic. Low dosages are viewed as helpful for several types of pain and inflammation. 50–200 mg three times a day is a good balance. For more flexibility in dosage, seek out a Traditional Chinese Medicine (TCM) practitioner.

White Willow Bark
The bark from the white willow and others in its species is the natural source for the anti-inflammatory properties found in aspirin (salicylic glycosides). It therefore comes as no surprise that willow bark has been used for thousands of years to treat all manner of pain and inflammation.

Being that it is a bark, to make it into a tea calls for a decoction process. You may also use powders mixed in liquid. Even though all of its medicinal properties have not been fully extracted in the powder form, pain reduction is still experienced.

Suggested dosage: Tincture, 10–20 drops as needed; tea, 1 teaspoon per cup.

Shiitake Mushrooms
Medicinal properties in mushrooms such as shiitake, maitake, and agaricus blazei have long been hailed for their health-promoting effects on chronic diseases like cancer. It therefore should come as no surprise that shiitake is now being recognized for its natural ability to inhibit inflammation. It contains unique nutrients that are hard to come by in a normal diet, such as ergothioneine, which obstructs oxidative stress.

Suggested dosage: 500 mg three times a day.

Cayenne Pepper (Capsaicin)
As a practitioner, I have mainly used this herb in the treatment of diabetic neuropathy (due to its ability to deplete nerve cells of substance P) and for poor circulation (and in some cases of weight loss). Capsaicin is the potent compound responsible for the hot taste of cayenne pepper, and is also a member of the nightshade family (discussed in Chapter 1). Substance P is an important factor in pain perception and, like other neuropeptides, can be released from the sensory nerve fibers found in the skin, muscle, and joints.

Cayenne also contains powerful antioxidants that protect the cells against the free radical damage which leads to inflammation. Quality is important, since this spice may be used often and exposing it to moisture will promote the production of mold. Be careful not to sprinkle herbs over hot steaming liquids or food while cooking.

Add cayenne to creams and lotions for external problems (such as on the lower extremities of people who suffer with diabetic neuropathy). Add it to hot liquids (according to taste tolerance) and on food. As a supplement, it can be purchased in capsules.

Suggested dosage: 100–200 mg three times a day.

Rhein (Rhubarb)
Because of the many negative outcomes associated with chronic and severe inflammation, there is currently a great demand for safe, effective remedies that treat inflammation. Of recent interest is the compound anthraquinone (rhein), which is derived from rhubarb and which has shown positive benefits for treatment of inflammatory symptoms. Products containing anthraquinone are now surfacing due to research underlining its inhibitory and anti-inflammatory role in the human body. Noni and aloe vera also contain anthraquinone properties.

Dosage will vary according to individual need. However, to give a general recommendation: tincture, 10–30 drops 2–3 times per day; powdered rhubarb root, 5–60 grains (about 1 teaspoon, up to 1/8 of an ounce); rhubarb seed, 20 grains of seed are equal to 30 grains of root powder, with the properties of the seeds being similar to those found in the root.

Skullcap (Scutellaria baicalensis)
Skullcap has been successfully used to treat a wide variety of problems, ranging from inflammation (especially involving nerve pain) to insomnia, anxiety, depression, migraines, and allergies. Inflammation of the nervous system often indicates unmet nutritional needs in the area being affected, or the health status of the whole person. Simply blocking nerve endings will not be enough to solve this problem, yet this is the method taken with prescription medication. Addressing nutritional requirements with extra supplementation should be a main consideration in order to quickly address all physiological factors. (Another herb with similar attributes is valerian, well known for its pain relieving and sedative properties).

Depending on the type of pain, lower dosages (10–15 drops) taken every 30–60 minutes may be more effective until pain becomes lessened.

In acute stages, 4 doses of 15 drops every 15 minutes over a 1–2 hour period would not be uncommon, with the dosage decreasing as symptoms subside. Otherwise, the suggested dosage is 15–25 drops of tincture 3–6 times a day.

Glycyrrhizin (Licorice Root Extract)
An active element found in licorice root, glycyrrhizin is most often taken for digestion and gut dysbiosis problems. In Chinese medicine, it has long been used to treat liver problems such as chronic hepatitis, liver tumors, and health maintenance of liver function.

As an anti-inflammatory agent, glycyrrhizin possesses a multitude of natural and very effective properties, along with anti-viral agents. Licorice is well known for its demulcent qualities, soothing inflamed mucous membranes of the lungs, throat, gastrointestinal tract and stomach. Other areas of benefit include a lessening of the symptoms of fibromyalgia and chronic fatigue.

Suggested dosage: decoction tea, 1 teaspoon per cup of water three times a day; liquid extract, 20–60 drops 1–4 times per day.

Ginger
Ginger has been used medicinally long before science developed an interest in its ability to treat inflammation and gastric problems. It contains as many as 500 different properties, only a few of which have been scientifically studied. Because ginger has strong antibacterial properties, it can help prevent colds and flu as well as treat their symptoms.

New research has also revealed that ginger is such a powerful anti-cancer medicine that it can kill 10,000 times as many cancer cells as chemotherapy when incorporated into your diet. My personal preference is grated fresh ginger root (of a mushy consistency) mixed with boiling water and raw honey. I also use it abundantly when cooking any Asian or Indian recipes, as well in soups and salad dressings and dishes comprised of a mixture of grains, legumes, and rice.

Garlic
This household staple has acquired an impressive healing profile. This is because garlic contains a potent agent called allicin, which has the capabil-

ity to destroy even the most antibiotic resistant strains of bacteria, making it a valuable anti-inflammatory. Use liberally in your food, preferably without destroying its medicinal properties by over-cooking, or purchase in supplement form and take as needed.

CHAPTER 10

Diet Therapy for Reversing Inflammation

WHEN SEEKING TO reduce chronic inflammation, the diet is a pivotal initial factor to consider. Diet is a major contributor to inflammation; that said, since there are so many diet considerations and variables to consider when dealing with specific health problems, diet suggestions must be attuned to individual needs. For instance, a diabetic's diet would not be the same as that of a person suffering with heart disease, arthritis, or inflammatory bowel disease.

All the same, there are common threads when it comes to the foods that either trigger inflammation or prevent it. The food choices recommended in this chapter are intended to focus on maximum nutrition and digestibility. Later in this chapter, you'll find easy meal suggestions to help reduce and prevent the onset of inflammation. Don't overlook the importance of your diet or put off changing your meal plans—you will be amazed at how much difference a simple change or two can make to your overall health and well-being.

Smoothies

Blended beverages are a one-stop way to provide extra nutrition while helping to reduce appetite and provide yourself with a feeling of fullness. These type of drinks let your creativity run wild, making combinations of ingredients that are not seen in stores. Another attractive feature is that smoothies provide an avenue for special health essentials without an unpleasant taste. They are wonderful for disguising foods or supplements that are missing in the diet but are still necessary for an individual's growth, function, and productivity. In other words, smoothies and blended drinks are perfect for the picky eaters in your family!

The following examples are but a few of the numerous possibilities available.

Popular Smoothie Ingredients

Almond milk	Fruit juice	Stevia (herb)
Cashew milk	Fruit fresh-frozen	Ginger (herb)
Coconut milk	Fruit dried	Mint family (herb)
Coconut cream	Fruit concentrates	Carob powder
Goat's milk	Berries	Cinnamon
Rice milk	Nuts	Vanilla
Sesame milk	Nut butter	Lemon
Soy milk	Seeds	Lime
Sunflower milk	Egg yolk	Cold pressed oils
Dairy milk	Avocado	Protein powder
Dairy cream	Agave	Yogurt
Ice cubes	Raw honey	Supplements
Water	Maple syrup	

Juicing

One of the biggest challenges we face when changing our diet is finding ways to feed our bodies more adequately. Drinking fresh juice is one of the most innovative therapies available to quell inflammation and help reverse even the deadliest of diseases. By taking better care of the body's nutritional requirements by regularly drinking quality juices, many complaints start to fall away.

Fresh-juiced liquids *are* a source of food in and of themselves; what's more, they can be enhanced to become meal replacements when you incorporate a variety of vegetables, essential fatty acids, and protein sources. What results is a meal that can fill many of the nutritional gaps that were currently unattainable through your daily diet. In addition to picking up vitamins and minerals, the body also receives an abundance of antioxidants and enzymes that may have been missing. These will become invaluable to your future health and longevity.

Partner Your Ingredients to Suit Your Digestion
If one were to investigate how their digestive system processes material, they would learn that vegetables and fruits should not be combined in the same juice formula. When eating a meal, fruit should be consumed 30 minutes prior to food or 2 hours following a meal (not immediately after). When eaten with a meal, fruit rots and ferments, causing gas, bloating, and indigestion. Indigestion is also caused from food combining (for example, eating starch and protein together). However, an apple to a large mixed vegetable juice formula seems to be acceptable by many professionals. What is not typically acceptable is multiple fruits, like strawberries, peaches, and melons, being mixed with carrots and beets. (Pure green juice mixed with a fruit works fine.)

Popular Juice Ingredients

Acai berry	Cilantro	Nut butters (cashew, almond, hemp)
Acerola cherry	Coconut	
Apple	Coconut milk	Olive oil (extra virgin)
Apricots	Collard greens	Onion (spring/scallion)
Aronia berry	Cranberry	Orange
Asparagus	Cucumber	Papaya
Avocado	Dandelion greens	Parsley
Beet and greens	Dates	Passion fruit
Bananas	Endive	Peach
Bee pollen	Fennel bulb	Peas (fresh from pods)
Bitter melon	Figs	Pear
Blackberry	Flax seed oil	Pepper (jalapeno)
Black cherry juice (whole)	Goji	Pepper (green)
	Grapes (purple or white)	Pepper (red)
Blueberry		Pineapple
Broccoli	Grapefruit	Plums
Brussels sprout	Kale	Pomegranate
Cabbage (green)	Kiwi	Potato
Cabbage (red)	Lemon	Radish
Camu camu	Lettuce (romaine)	Raspberry
Carrot	Lime	Spinach
Cauliflower	Lychee	Sprouts (barley, broccoli, alfalfa)
Celery	Mango	
Chia oil	Melon (cantaloupe)	Strawberry

Sweet potato   Tomato   Wheat grass
Tahini   Watermelon   Wolfberry
Tangerine   Wheat germ

Spices
Ginger   Mint family   Cinnamon
Black pepper   Algae   Garlic
Fresh basil   Kelp   Pink salt
Cayenne pepper   Dulse   Pumpkin pie spice
Turmeric   Pure vanilla   Quality cocoa powder
Apple cider vinegar Carob powder

Juice Preparation
Prepare fruits and vegetables as you would normally, removing the skin, rind, and seeds before juicing or blending. If the skin on the fruit or vegetable is normally eaten, do not peel before juicing. For blended drinks and smoothies, you may choose to add ice cubes or liquids to lighten up the consistency of the formula.

Health drinks are an opportunity to add special ingredients that, while they may be disguised, will really boost the immune's inflammation response and nutritional value. Consider supplements that are in powder form or capsules that can be opened up. Essential fatty acids are perfect, as are probiotic powders or fresh cultures. Spices like turmeric and ginger fight inflammation and are equipped with antiviral properties while aiding digestion. Acai, goji, and wolfberries are extremely rich in superior antioxidants that protect the cells in our body and significantly lower inflammation.

Green Juices
Green juice preparation and formulas often differ from conventional vegetable juice recipes. The volume consumed is usually far less (depending on accompanying ingredients). The base is the biggest difference, as carrots are usually the primary ingredient contributing to the bulk of a vegetable formula.

Green juice concentrate amounts to a couple of ounces in volume, and is often supplemented with fruit and spices. Lemon and lime are two favorite ingredients, and can counter bitter tastes without needing to add a sweetener.

Wheat Grass
Concentrated juice from green plants like wheatgrass, kale, parsley, watercress, cilantro, dandelion, barley, and sprouts are all very potent in terms of nutrition and in taste. Usually when ingesting these green juices, less is more. The amount of wheat grass juiced and consumed at one time generally amounts to 2–3 ounces. Greens like dandelion or parsley would normally be consumed in far smaller quantities, more often accompanied by other vegetables or fruit.

Juice or blended formulas using greens as the base are normally simple recipes and are not complicated unless you feel adventurous or really desire a different taste. People who are advocates of green concentrated juices are more interested in their health and well-being and far more inclined to put up with an off-putting taste. Having said that, if the experience is so unpleasant to the point of not continuing with green juicing, alter the formula to enable its consumption using sweeter vegetables or fruit. See the recipes included in chapter 11 for some examples of simple formulas that have a tremendous impact on inflammation while being quick and easy to make.

Adding Protein to Liquids
Vegetable and green juice formulas should be your primary consideration in picking up mineral shortages. Fruit juices are energizing, while smoothies are often prepared as a meal substitute.

This is not to say that vegetable- and fruit-based liquids cannot be nutritionally equivalent to a protein based smoothie, in order to be considered a balanced meal. To start formulating a complete meal preparation, protein powders are an excellent complement to your juice formula. Protein adds dietary balance and helps retain the feeling of satiety. Remember that protein must be present when taking any supplements containing minerals in order to ensure optimum absorption. A few favorites include hemp powder, rice bran powder, whey powders (whey is now available lactose free), goat's whey and pea powder.

Other sources include egg yolk, nut butters, seeds, amino acid powders, cottage cheese, yogurt or kefir, powdered algae, and edible yeast (including nutritional flaked yeast, Tortula, Engevita, and Brewers).

Dietary Fiber
Misconceptions still exist today surrounding the role of dietary fiber. Viewed mainly as a constipation aid, these preconceived notions of fiber

greatly limit its use and the wonderful benefits it has to offer. Fiber benefits us nutritionally and can be utilized to aid a variety of health problems. For instance, fiber helps control inflammation by diluting inflammatory substances and assists in their removal from the body. Certain types of plant fiber also possess natural anti-inflammatories, in addition to its nutritional content.

Another benefit of fiber is its ability to slow down the absorption of sugar and carbohydrates while also keeping fats from being reabsorbed into the body. If you require fat and sugar levels to be lowered, take fiber with every meal as well as in your juice preparations.

Good fiber choices include ground flax seeds, psyllium husks, locust bean, guar gum, rice bran, oat bran, and pectin, all of which are highly absorbable and gentle on the gastrointestinal system.

Pro-Inflammatory Sweeteners

Since man first became introduced to the sweet things in life, he has sought after it with increasing determination. In today's commercial market, pro-inflammatory corn syrup (high fructose corn syrup) is constantly gaining ground, replacing refined sugar (which is a potent pro-inflammatory) in many manufactured products.

High fructose corn syrup was invented by Japanese researchers as an inexpensive sweetener for soft drinks, and is six times sweeter than sugar. Unfortunately, corn syrup has since become subsided by the government and is found in many commercial products, including breads, cereals, ketchup, and soft drinks. It is added to a wide variety of foods and during food preparation to make food taste better.

Corn syrup is not recommended for anyone who has inflammation, especially for those with a compromised digestive system or disease. One of the issues with fructose in relation to gut problems is that this form of sugar is not well absorbed through the intestinal tract, and becomes a food source for yeast, fungus, and other intestinal microbes. What results is damage to the lining of intestines (gut permeability) and stomach, setting the gut up for chronic inflammation.

Other problems associated with higher consumption of fructose include liver dysfunction and an imbalance of lipids and triglycerides that influences heart anomalies.

As a note of interest, glucose and fructose do not fall into the same category as being a necessary food supply. Intravenous glucose can sustain life, whereas intravenous fructose cannot.

Natural Fruit Sugar
The natural sugar found in fruits is of a much lower concentration than manufactured products, and retains all the health benefits provided by the vitamins, minerals, antioxidants, enzymes and fiber. The form of sugar contained in fruit is a complex carbohydrate, which has a much slower release than refined sugar (a simple carbohydrate). The fiber in fruit is the deciding factor in this, as fiber traps the sugar molecules in the intestines after digestion, providing an additional forty-five minutes of glucose (food) to the brain. Sucrose (refined sugar) does not process via the liver and goes directly into the blood stream within fifteen minutes.

Additional Healthy Sweeteners
When a sweeter taste is called for, natural sweeteners may be added to your healthy juice formulas or food. At times when healthy drinks do not contain any fruit or vegetables that have a sweet taste, or when green concentrates need extra help in order to encourage some individuals to drink them, try adding small amounts of honey, stevia (herb), palm sugar, date sugar, agave, molasses, or maple syrup.

Depending on the type of drink or juice being made, other options include reconstituted (soaked) dried fruit like dates, prunes, figs, and raisins. Pineapple and grape juice are wonderful for covering the strong flavors of leafy greens or less sweet fruit formulas.

Daily Meal Plan for Reversing Inflammation

The majority of people have not been taught how to eat properly—that is, according to our physiological needs. Addressing the diet, as we have said, is the most impactful way to reduce the influence of physical and emotional stressors.

What follows is my simplified daily eating plan for eating in the right balance that coincides to the pH balance of our blood and the body's digestive processes. One of the goals for eating proportionately is to avoid stimulating the parathyroid gland into robbing calcium from our bones and tissues in order to maintain a proper pH blood ratio. An imbalance occurs when the daily intake of food is more acidic (meat, dairy, starch, grains, and white potatoes) compared to alkaline foods (most fruits, vegetables, and alkaline dairy such as yogurt, kefir, and whey powder).

This eating plan will also contribute to weight loss, if needed; otherwise, eat more of whatever you like as detailed below, as long as you aim for proper combinations.

General Rules
Our digestive system is not set up to cope with large amounts of starch and protein consumed at one time. Yet most people are raised on exactly such a diet. This way of eating automatically reduces the level of nutrition that is most required by our bodies, hinders the maintenance of proper pH blood levels, and restricts the body from assimilating nutrients. If you fill up on the heavy starch and protein foods, there will also be very little room for your body's desired intake of vegetables. To top things off, many people finish off their meals with a dessert that is usually made of pro-inflammatory ingredients.

The good news is that by simply not combining food and by incorporating more vegetables in place of starch components, you will substantially raise the level of nutrition in your meal, enhance digestibility, and not lose a bit of your daily energy. This is especially noticeable for anyone sitting during the afternoon, whether in a classroom or an office, following a lunch that consisted of meat and pasta or bread.

Avoid reaching for easy fixes during the midday slump! Between 2:30 and 3:30 in the afternoon, we are all normally a bit more sluggish. It is at this time of day that our thyroid gland reaches its lowest point. People normally gravitate to a sugar or carbohydrate fix. Protein and/or fruit will serve you far better, and will allow you to avoid the spike and drop of blood sugar levels.

On that note, be sure to feed your thyroid gland! It requires a small amount of iodine daily in order to make thyroid hormone. Inexpensive liquid iodine drops can be purchased at all health related stores that sell supplements. (Please refer to Chapter 6 for a list of nutrients that are routinely missing from modern diets.)

> **A Few Personal Diet Recommendations**
>
> Even I find it hard to eat the amount of raw food recommended for our biochemical makeup. Vegetable juice or green juice is an easy way to add more raw food into your diet. I started vegetable juicing in my late twenties, and I have never experienced a sluggish workday. I also eat less on those days.
>
> I typically have cooked beans on hand for their fiber and protein content. They are the best for binding to fat and to slow down sugar absorption. I also make frequent use of dried beans (soaking and cooking them); the ones I most often use are red, black, and yellow-eyed beans. I usually eat a small amount around each meal.
>
> As a final note: even if you are trying to eat properly, it doesn't mean you can't occasionally have a cheat day. There are times in the year, such as the holiday season, where I find myself making traditional meals. I may know that I am not going to feel good that week as a result; however, we're only human. Looking at the relationship between food and the biochemical nature of our digestive systems means that a new way of eating can quickly became a habit. If you can get used to feeling good and retaining your energy, you'll find that you desire cheat days less and less.

The following are a list of recommendations that form the backbone of this natural inflammation reversal protocol.

Cooking Process: Do not overcook your vegetables; this prevents the destruction of the antioxidant and enzymatic activity, along with other phytochemicals. Do not overheat or burn your food, and do not use cooking oils that promote inflammation and disease.

Processed Foods: Eliminate all processed foods from your diet and replace them with whole (ideally organic) food that you purchase and cook yourself.

Protein: Choose lean, low-fat flesh proteins such as lamb, chicken, fish, seafood and vegetarian protein choices.

Leafy Greens and Sprouts: Create a habit of eating more of these health-promoting and inflammation-busting foods. Even if you feel you do not have enough appetite for a whole salad, a handful of sprouts or mixed greens makes a great addition to your meal.

Vegetables: Widen your variety of vegetable intake in terms of color and texture. Stretch your taste buds and try something different from the traditional items we become accustomed to from our youth.

Fruits: Fruit isn't as hard a sell as vegetables, since most people like the sweet things in life. But there are so many spectacular choices available today from all over the world that offer far greater amounts of antioxidants and carotenoids than the common apple, pear, and strawberry. Try fruits that make for a great accompaniment to a salad, such as mango, lychee, and dragon fruit.

Spices: Widen your familiarity with the spices that may be used in everyday cooking. Experiment and have fun with different flavors, using them liberally on a daily basis. If your food is typically plain or heavily salted, you may want guidance and ideas from friends or the numerous recipes online and in books to help wake up your taste buds. When it comes to inflammation-reducing antioxidants, herbs and spices are significantly higher than most other foods on a proportionate basis.

Extra Dietary Supplementation: Take supplements just before you eat your meals unless otherwise indicated by product brands.

Fiber: For adequate fiber content, add either 2 tablespoons of ground flax seeds to liquid just before you eat or have $1/3$ cup of cooked beans with or after the meal.

Diet Therapy for Reversing Inflammation

Daily Menu Plan

The following is meant to serve as a guide; feel free to replace with foods you like as long as you do not combine starch and protein together. Keep protein and starch foods in small portions and increase vegetables and fruit intake. Drink liquid chlorophyll and water throughout the day, as well as herbal teas.

BREAKFAST	2 cups of vegetable juice or fruit juice, with the addition of protein powder, ground flax seeds, flax seed oil, nutritional flaked yeast, and any other supplements may be added or taken separately.
	Fresh fruit smoothie
	1 cup yogurt (plain, organic, or Greek) topped with nuts, seeds and fresh fruit; may drizzle with raw honey.
	Steel cut oatmeal, Red River cereal, quinoa, GMO-free corn flakes, or other gluten-free cereals (low in sugar)
MID-MORNING	Fruit: Can be eaten between breakfast and lunch.
	When vegetable juice becomes a breakfast habit, you may notice yourself being far less hungry throughout the morning, and your lunch could become lighter, as well.
LUNCH	One or two of the following suggestions (manage portion size):
	• Salad with a small amount of dressing; try flax seed oil mixed with lemon juice or apple cider vinegar, herbs, seasoning, raw honey
	• Tuna salad or egg salad, eaten by itself or with a salad
	• Rye crisp with thinly sliced old cheese or rice crackers (or similar low-calorie starch) with peanut butter or other nut butters
	• Vegetable wrap (gluten free wrap)
	• Homemade soup
	• Plain yogurt and fruit drizzled with raw honey
	• Raw vegetables (as much as you desire)

MID-DAY	One or two of the following suggestions: • 1 handful of almonds or walnuts • 1 small bunch of grapes, berries or other fruits; or protein drink • Raw carrots, cucumbers, peppers, or other similar vegetables • Yogurt • Freshly made vegetable, green, or fresh fruit juice
DINNER	**Option 1** 4 ounces lean meat or fish 3 vegetables (green, yellow, red, or orange; no potatoes, pasta, or bread) Salad • Legumes mixed with grains, vegetables and herbs. • Stir fry with noodles or rice (lots of veggies, small amount of protein) **Option 2** 1–2 cups of cooked gluten-free pasta with tomato sauce (lots of herbs) or pesto (no meat, fish, bread) Green vegetables (large portion) Salad Zucchini pasta or spaghetti squash, with a protein proportionate to the individual, garnished with tomato sauce or oil and herbs. **Option 3** 1 cup cooked wild and brown rice (cooked in broth or water) OR Quinoa, millet, and amaranth cooked together. Combine with 1 cup cooked legumes (lentils or beans), sautéed onions (caramelized), garlic, herbs, and other vegetables (no flesh protein or starch such as bread, potatoes or pasta).

	Option 4 Hearty soup with whole grains and legumes. Soups that incorporate all aspects of a balanced meal are wonderful for dinner or lunch. They may even resemble a stew, which is another great meal suggestion. **Option 5** Vegetarian lasagna made with layers of sweet potato, zucchini, and Sicilian eggplant. Precook sweet potatoes, slice and lightly cook other vegetables. Cover each vegetable layer with your favorite tomato sauce and cheese. The cooking procedure is the same as for traditionally made lasagna. Remember to add your favorite aromatic herbs like garlic, basil, and oregano.
SNACKS	• Apple, or ½–1 cup pineapple • Raw vegetables • Citrus fruit • Melons (not mixed with other fruits) • Air popped popcorn • Small handful of nuts or seeds
BEVERAGES	• Freshly made juice: vegetable juice, green juice, fruit juice • Liquid chlorophyll in water throughout the day • Tea • Fermented drinks • Coffee substitutes

CHAPTER 11

Recipes

ANTI-INFLAMMATORY COCKTAILS

The type of juicer used in the following juice recipes separates the pulp from the juice. Remember that all fresh juices should be consumed within an hour of being made.

Michelle Honda's Favorite Vegetable Juice

2 pounds carrots
1 medium beet
1 apple (optional)
6 dandelion leaves
6 sprigs parsley

Follow the instructions for your juicer and combine all ingredients.

Immune Booster

1 pound carrots
3 kale leaves
1 cup spinach
2 teaspoons wheat grass juice
1 cup broccoli sprouts

Follow the instructions for your juicer and combine all ingredients.

Inflammation Buster

6 large kale leaves
½ bunch spinach
6 sprigs parsley
6 sprigs cilantro
1 medium cucumber
2 sweet apples
½ lime
½ teaspoon grated ginger
1 tablespoon raw honey

Follow the instructions for your juicer and combine all ingredients.

Energy Booster

1 medium beet
2 sweet apples
4 leaves Swiss chard
4 leaves kale or beet greens
½ lemon juiced
1 medium cucumber
6 sprigs parsley
3 mint leaves
1 teaspoon turmeric powder
1 teaspoon algae powder (blue or green)
1 tablespoon raw honey or favorite sweetener

Follow the instructions for your juicer and combine all ingredients.

Morning Delight

4 oranges, peeled
5 dandelion leaves
5 kale leaves
6 mint leaves
¼ teaspoon cinnamon

Follow the instructions for your juicer and combine all ingredients. Sweeten to taste with stevia, raw honey or agave.

Wheat Grass/Kale Juice

½ ounces wheat grass juice
1 ounce kale juice

Follow the instructions for your juicer and combine all ingredients.

Wheat Grass/Lemon/Ginger Juice

2 ounces wheat grass juice
¼ lemon, juiced
½ inch fresh ginger
1 teaspoon raw honey

Follow the instructions for your juicer and combine all ingredients.

Wheat Grass/Orange/Lemon Balm Leaves Juice

2 ounces wheat grass
12 lemon balm leaves
1 orange, peeled
Optional/mint or peppermint leaves

Follow the instructions for your juicer and combine all ingredients.

Wheat Grass/Lemon/Cilantro Juice

2 ounces wheat grass
1 ounce freshly squeezed lemon
4 sprigs cilantro
1 teaspoon raw honey

Follow the instructions for your juicer and combine all ingredients.

Wheat Grass Combo

2 ounces wheat grass
3 apples cored with the skin on
5 kale leaves
½ lemon, juiced
Optional: ¼ teaspoon fresh grated ginger or 6 mint or lemon balm leaves

Follow the instructions for your juicer and combine all ingredients.

FRUIT JUICE RECIPES

Apricot/Pear/Peach Juice

4 apricots
2 peaches
1 pear
1 apple
Ginger, to taste

Blend or juice all ingredients. Finely grate ¼ teaspoon fresh ginger and add to a blender type juicer, or ⅛ inch slice of fresh ginger to a juicer that separates the pulp.

Aronia/Apple/Pear Juice

2 cups aronia berries
2 sweet apples
2 pears
3 drops pure vanilla

Blend or juice all ingredients.

Blueberry/Cherry/Plum/Apple/Pear Juice

2 cups blueberries
2 cups Bing or acerola cherries
2 sweet apples
2 purple plums
1 pear
¼ lemon juiced
1 teaspoon raw honey
Cinnamon or favorite spice

Blend or juice all ingredients.

Strawberry/Pineapple/Grape Juice

2 cups strawberries
2 cups purple, green, or red grapes (seedless)
1 cup chopped pineapple
(Optional) ¼ cup Acai juice or ½ cup berries

Blend or juice all ingredients.

Mango/Banana/Lychee/Wolfberry Juice

2 mangos or papaya
1 banana
12 lychee fruit, prepared
¼ cup dried wolfberries
1 orange peeled

Blend or juice all ingredients.

Passion Fruit/Peach/Lemon Juice

4 passion fruit, prepared
2 peaches or 3 apricots
1 small lemon, juiced
(Optional) mint leaves
1 tablespoon raw honey or sweetener of choice

Blend or juice all ingredients.

Black Cherry/Pineapple/Peach Juice

2 cups black cherries (pit removed) *or* 1 cup juice
  or (¼ cup concentrate to ¾ cup water)
1 cup pineapple chunks
2 peaches

Blend or juice all ingredients.

Apple/Pomegranate/Kale/Dandelion Juice

3 apples
1 cup pomegranate juice
4 kale leaves
3 dandelion leaves

Blend or juice all ingredients. Sweeten with stevia, agave or raw honey to taste.

BLENDED DRINKS AND SMOOTHIE RECIPES

Michelle Honda's Favorite Smoothie Recipe

2 cups coconut milk
8 ice cubes
1 large ripe banana
½ cup strawberries or blueberries
½ cup fresh pineapple
2 ounces hemp powder
1 tablespoon carob powder
2 tablespoons flax seed oil
1 tablespoon nutritional flaked yeast
1 teaspoon probiotic powder
(Optional) 2 teaspoons raw honey

Blend ingredients together in a blender to desired consistency.

Tahini/Pineapple Smoothie

½ cup organic yogurt
1 cup pineapple, cubed
1 cup water or 8 ice cubes
2 tablespoons sesame seed butter (Tahini)
1 teaspoon lemon juice
2 tablespoons raw honey or agave

Blend ingredients together in a blender to desired consistency.

Nutrition Packed Smoothie

2 cups liquid of choice (milk replacement, fruit juice, or milk)
1 avocado
1 large ripe banana
8 ice cubes
2 ounces whey powder or (hemp, goat's whey*, or pea powder)
1 tablespoon nutritional flaked yeast
1 teaspoon bee pollen
1 raw egg yolk
2 tablespoon lecithin granules
1 tablespoon wheat germ
2 drops of iodine or seaweed powder like dulse or kelp
2 tablespoons raw honey or sweetener of choice
(Optional) 1 tablespoon cocoa powder
*Whey powder is available lactose-free.

Blend ingredients together in a blender to desired consistency.

Note: Coconut milk is not recommended in this recipe due to its high calorie content. However, if weight gain is required, then coconut milk or cream is a good choice.

Black Cherry/Orange Smoothie

¼ cup black cherry concentrate
1 cup pineapple juice
2 oranges
1 cup organic yogurt
2 tablespoons raw honey or agave
Optional/ice cubes

Blend ingredients together in a blender to desired consistency.

Date/Nut Smoothie

4 pitted dates
¼ cup almond butter
1 banana
2 cups milk of choice

Blend ingredients together in a blender to desired consistency.

Prune/Nut Milk/Banana Smoothie

6 prunes, pitted
1 cup milk of choice
1 tablespoon nut butter
1 small banana
(Optional) 1 teaspoon cocoa powder

Blend ingredients together in a blender to desired consistency.

Molasses/Nut Milk Drink

1 cup milk of choice
1 tablespoon organic black strap molasses
1 tablespoon nut butter

Blend ingredients together in a blender to desired consistency.

Pomegranate/Grape Drink

2–3 pomegranates
2 cups grapes
½ cup protein powder of choice

First, add fruits to a juicer that removes the seeds or use a food processor and strain seeds. Then blend ingredients together in a blender to desired consistency.

Protein/Fruit Drink

1 cup fruit juice of choice
1 ounce whey powder
1 egg yolk
¼ teaspoon kelp or dulse powder

Blend ingredients together in a blender to desired consistency.

Coconut/Fig Drink

1 cup coconut milk
4 fresh figs or reconstituted dried figs

Blend ingredients together in a blender to desired consistency.

Avocado/Seed Drink

½ avocado
1 cup vegetable juice, fruit juice, or milk of choice*
1 tablespoon seed meal or butter
1 teaspoon raw honey or maple syrup

Blend ingredients together in a blender to desired consistency.

SOUPS AND SALADS

The following recipes provide light examples of dishes that favor nutrition while reducing inflammation.

Cabbage and Bitter Greens

2 cups shredded Savoy cabbage
2 cups dandelion leaves, chopped
2 cups Belgian endive
½ cup sweet white or red onion
1 tablespoon parsley chopped

Dressing

½ cup freshly squeezed lemon juice
1 tablespoon apple cider vinegar
3 tablespoons flax seed oil or hemp oil
¼ teaspoon kelp powder or pink salt
⅛ teaspoon freshly ground black powder
1 tablespoon hemp hearts
2 teaspoons agave syrup
¼ teaspoon freshly minced garlic

Toss all salad ingredients together and add dressing. Mix until evenly coated. Sprinkle with a hard cheese or crumble feta cheese on top, if desired.

Broccoli and Carrot Salad

3 cups broccoli florets
1 cup coarsely grated carrot
½ cup diced sweet white onion
2 tablespoons dried organic cranberries, chopped
½ cup coarsely chopped walnuts
⅓ cup low fat mayonnaise
2 teaspoons agave syrup
¼ teaspoon pink salt

Combine all ingredients. Add dressing and toss until well blended.

Creamy Dairy Free Celery Soup

1 quart low sodium chicken broth
8 large celery stalks, chopped
1 large white potato, peeled and diced
1 cup diced sweet white onion
1 large garlic clove, minced
½ teaspoon pink salt
¼ cup butter

In a heavy bottomed saucepan, using low heat, sauté onions, celery, and garlic in butter to soften. Do not brown.

Pour in chicken broth. Add diced potato and salt. Cook until the potatoes are soft.

Once cooled, add to a blender. I do not blend the whole soup into a cream (but you can if you'd like to). The first half is blended until creamy; the second half is blended on low to retain small pieces of celery and vegetable matter. Add black pepper upon serving.

DINNER

Braised Halibut

2. 4–6 ounces firm fish (halibut, haddock, sea bass, or salmon)
1 large sweet potato
2 cups freshly grated zucchini
Seasoned oil for brushing on fish
1 tablespoon butter
1 tablespoon brown sugar
Extra virgin olive oil
Fresh chives for garnish

Bake or microwave sweet potato. Once cooked, remove skin and mash.

Have grated zucchini prepared and ready to be cooked once the fish has been put on the grill. Brush fish with extra virgin olive oil and season with lemon, pink salt, pepper and parsley.

Add butter, brown sugar, and grated zucchini to a heavy bottomed pan. Sautee on medium to higher heat until the mixture starts to wilt. Do not overcook the zucchini.

To plate, add an oval mound of sweet potato and zucchini beside one another. Place the fish on top of the zucchini round and sprinkle fresh chives on top. The highlight of this dish is your favorite fish braised on the grill paired with a layer of mashed sweet potato and sautéed grated zucchini.

Raw Tomato Sauce

If you have never made raw tomato sauce, you are in for a treat. It is lighter, yet the flavors are far more pungent. Naturally you are not losing any flavor due to cooking; therefore, the amount of garlic and herbs as compared to cooked versions is considerably less.

Another main difference is the water content in the sauce. To produce a thicker sauce, blend your skinless and seedless fresh tomatoes in a blender and let drip through a gauze cloth or very fine sieve to remove a portion of the tomato water. Otherwise, blend all ingredients together and pour over hot pasta. On a personal note, I have not felt the need to strain tomato water; however, it may depend on your desired usage.

Raw tomato sauce is suitable for intestinal problems involving inflammation, unless there is chronic diarrhea or bleeding occurring. In such cases, easily digestible alkaline foods are required, whereas cooked tomato sauce would be too acidic.

6 cups chopped, skinless and seedless fresh tomatoes

1 large garlic clove

2 tablespoons freshly chopped basil

1 tablespoon freshly chopped parsley

2 tablespoons extra virgin olive oil

1 scallion, chopped

1 tablespoon raw honey

¼ teaspoon pink salt

Option: oregano

In a blender or food processor, coarsely blend (if you like texture; otherwise, it will resemble a lighter-colored tomato puree). Pour over your favorite grain or vegetable pasta.

Eggplant Cutlets

1 large round Sicilian eggplant (whitish-purple), sliced into ¼ inch rounds
Gluten free flour or all purpose flour
2 eggs
1¼ cups gluten free bread crumbs
¼ cup almond meal
Oil (for cooking)

Coat the eggplant rounds in flour. Whisk the eggs together, and then dip the floured eggplant into the egg bath. Blend together bread crumbs and almond meal, and coat eggplant with the mixture. Using extra virgin olive oil (or coconut oil) as needed, sauté on *low* heat to ensure thorough cooking of eggplant without over-browning.

Fresh Pesto Sauce

Pesto is another raw sauce that is more often made with basil as the primary ingredient. I have made this sauce with only parsley and found it suited many people's palates, even those that are not fond of a strong basil flavor. As with the above sauce, consider how much flavor you normally prefer.

3 cups fresh basil leaves
½ cup extra virgin olive oil
3 garlic cloves
¼ teaspoon pink salt
½ cup parsley leaves (optional)
½ cup whole walnut halves
½ cup grated parmesan cheese
¼ teaspoon red pepper flakes

In a food processor, combine the olive oil, garlic, salt and red pepper flakes. Blend thoroughly. Add the basil and parsley leaves and blend to desired consistency. Once blended, coarsely grind the walnuts. I suggest stirring in the grated cheese after the noodles and pesto sauce have been well mixed. Add additional cheese upon serving to suit individual taste. Serve immediately.

Fruit Gel Dessert (Agar)

Agar is a vegetable gelatin derived from seaweed, with only 3 calories per gram. It is odorless and tasteless, and can be purchased in the form of powder, bars or flakes. Look for Agar in natural food stores and Asian grocery stores.

There are endless flavor possibilities and many applications. Agar can be used to make jelly candies using sweetened milk or fruit juice, gelatin cocktail shots, or various desserts and fillings, and can be added to juice, coffee, teas, milk and milk substitutes, and even broths for a different treat.

Ratio:
- One bar is equivalent to 2 teaspoons of Agar powder.
- 2 tablespoons of Agar flakes is approximant to 2 teaspoons of Agar powder.
- To thicken 1 cup of liquid, use 1 teaspoon Agar powder, 1 tablespoon Agar flakes, or ½ Agar bar. Depending on desired firmness, use less or more agar.

Certain fruits contain enzymes that may prevent gelling, such as pineapples, papaya, mangos, citrus, and peaches. When a sweeter taste is called for, choose stevia, agave syrup or raw honey.

3 cups unsweetened grape juice
3 teaspoons agar powder
1½ cups mixed fruit of choice

Place juice in a saucepan and mix in agar powder and any desired sweeteners. Bring to a boil and simmer for about 5–10 minutes. Transfer to preferred container and chill for approximately 45 minutes (until the gel starts to set). Fold in fruit and chill until firm.

CONCLUSION

OVER THE COURSE of this book, we've been taken on an inflammation journey, learning to understand and appreciate its processes and manifestations in our bodies. Inflammation has been shown to be both our best friend and worst adversary, all dependent on whether our diet and lifestyle is in sync with our innate nature. Likewise, we have seen how medication can adversely affect our inflammation and detoxification pathways and the consequences of their prolonged usage.

But most important of all, we've seen that there is a better way!

The need for mainstream medications *can* be replaced with safe, natural solutions. As we've seen, the impact of our day-to-day dietary intake is one of the primary contributors to controlling inflammation and the spread of disease. By removing common culprits like toxic cooking oils and boosting key systems through judicious supplementation of vitamins and trace minerals, a person can begin a healing and disease reversal process.

And it *is* a process. But by understanding the many causes and imbalances in our day-to-day life, we gain the power to avert many of the negative outcomes of prolonged suffering. In knowing the cause for many mainstream disease complaints, you are now better equipped with information and solutions that can become part of your daily routine.

Even just making better food choices and changing out old habits for new ones will make a world of difference. Employing foods that lower inflammation—as opposed to those that enhance it—is an important first step. Add in anti-inflammatory supplements that will also promote a nutritionally sound body (like omega-3 fatty acids and fresh juice) and you're halfway there! And for those who need extra help in dealing with severe pain and inflammation, comfort can be provided through natural medicine and specific dietary nutrients, tailored to suit individual needs.

As a final note: the procedures and protocols in this book are intended to guide you through your healing process. But let's not forget the importance and benefits of prevention! Even upon being healed, we must remember that we do not want a repeat performance. Take advantage of all that you have learned to not only repair but maintain your body's energy levels. Take hold of your renewed energy as you move forward from this day on!

RESOURCES

Herbal Remedies: Additional Research Resources

54 Herb Society Forum
www.network54.com

Natural Standards Database
http://3rdparty.naturalstandard.com/frameset.asp

Cochrane Database Systems Reviews
http://community.cochrane.org/editorial-and-publishing-policy-resource/cochrane-database-systematic-reviews-cdsr

National Institutes of Health
https://nccih.nih.gov/

The National Institutes of Health (NIH) is a biomedical research facility primarily located in Bethesda, Maryland. An agency of the United States Department of Health and Human Services, it is the primary agency of the United States government responsible for biomedical and health-related research. The NIH both conducts its own scientific research through its Intramural Research Program (IRP) and provides major biomedical research funding to non-NIH research facilities through its Extramural Research Program.

National Institutes of Health Office of Dietary Supplements
http://ods.od.nih.gov/

National Center for Complementary and Alternative Medicine
https://nccih.nih.gov/

Natural Database Therapeutic Research
http://naturaldatabase.therapeuticresearch.com/home.aspx?cs=&s=ND

Herbs-at-a-Glance
https://nccih.nih.gov/health/herbsataglance.htm

Ayurvedic Medicine
https://nccih.nih.gov/health/ayurveda/introduction.htm

American Botanical Council ABC
http://abc.herbalgram.org/site/PageServer

American Herbalists Guild
http://www.americanherbalistsguild.com/

The College of Practitioners of Phytotherapy
http://www.phytotherapists.org/

Herb Research Foundation
http://www.herbs.org/herbnews/

International Herb Association
http://www.iherb.org/

National Institute of Medical Herbalists
http://www.nimh.org.uk/

Herbs are Special
http://www.herbsarespecial.com

Herbal and Supplement Sources

ACS (www.allcosmeticsource.com)

Eclectic Institute (www.eclectichrtb.com)

Frontier Co-op (http://www.frontiercoop.com/ourproducts.php)

Herb Pharm (www.herbpharm.com)

Natural Factors (www.naturalfactors.com)

Now Foods (www.nowfoods.com)

Nutraceutical Solaray (www.nutraceutical.com/collections/healthy/solaray)

Seroyal Genestra Professional Products (www.seroyal.com)

Vitamin Shoppe (www.vitaminshoppe.com)

BIBLIOGRAPHY

Introduction
1. Chris L. Peterson and Rachel Burton, "US Health Care Spending Comparison with Other OECD Countries," CRS Report for Congress, September 17, 2007, http://assets.opencrs.com/rpts/RL34175_20070917.pdf (accessed 01, 25, 2016).
2. Jeff Schweitzer, Inflammatory Claims About Inflammation. 05,29,2015.
3. American Gastroenterological Association. "Patient Center: NSAIDS." April 2010. http://www.gastro.org/patient-center/diet-medications/non-steriodal-anti-inflammatory-drugs-nsaids

Chapter 1
1. Zoltan P. Rona, Reversing Chronic Inflammation: Vitality Magazine, November 2012.
2. Tosi F1, Sartori F, Guarini P, Olivieri O, Martinelli N. Delta-5 and delta-6 desaturases: crucial enzymes in polyunsaturated fatty acid-related pathways with pleiotropic influences in health and disease. Adv Exp Med Biol. 2014;824:61-81. PMID: 25038994 DOI: 10.1007/978-3-319-07320-0_7
3. Jain, R. Sharma, A. Gupta, S. Sarethy, I. P. Gabrani, R. (2011). Solanum nigrum: current perspectives on therapeutic properties. Altern Med Rev, 16(1), 78-85.
5. Luigi Ferrucci… Relationship of Plasma Polyunsaturated Fatty Acids to Circulating Inflammatory Markers. J Clin. Endocrinol Metab, 2006 Feb: 91(2): 439-46, Epub 2005, Oct.18.

Chapter 2
1. Dr. Dwight Lundell, "Heart surgeon speaks out on what really causes heart disease." Prevent Disease. March 1, 2012.
2. Fran Balkwill. Cancer Research UK-funded research Inflammation Microenvironment 2013.
3. Safia Danovi. Feeling the heat – the link between inflammation and cancer Category: Science blog February 1, 2013
4. Psaila, B., & Lyden, D. (2009). The metastatic niche: adapting the foreign soil Nature Reviews Cancer, 9 (4), 285-293 DOI: 10.1038/nrc2621

5. Chong AY, Lupsa BC, Cochran EK, Gorden P. Efficacy of leptin therapy in the different forms of human lipodystrophy. Diabetologia. 2010;53:27–35.PubMed

6. Walsh, W. PhD, Metallothionein Deficiency in Autism Spectrum Disorders, 2002

7. Zoroglu SS, Armutcu F, Ozen S, et al. Increased oxidative stress and altered activities of erythrocyte free radical scavenging enzymes in autism. Eur Arch Psychiatry Clin Neurosci. 2004;254:143-147.

8 McBride J, Plant Pigments paint a rainbow of antioxidants. Agricultural Research. 11,1,1996

9. Katherine Esposito, MD, Raffaele Marfella MD, PhD. Effect of a Mediterranean-Style Diet on Endothelial Dysfunction and Markers of Vascular Inflammation in the Metabolic Syndrome. September 22/29, 2004

10. Leila Azadbakht, et al. "Beneficial Effects of a Dietary Approach to Stop Hypertension Eating Plan on Features of the Metabolic Syndrome," Diabetes Care 28(2005):2823-2831

11. M. Gonza´lez, M del Mar Bibiloni, Inflammatory markers and metabolic syndrome among adolescents. European Journal of Clinical Nutrition (2012), 1–5 & 2012 Macmillan Publishers Limited. June 2012

12. Phytother Res. 2005 Jun;19(6):530-7. Treating intermittent allergic rhinitis: a prospective, randomized, placebo and antihistamine-controlled study of Butterbur extract Ze 339. Schapowal A; Study Group.

Chapter 3

1. Reference: Omega 6 ratio to Omega 3 oils USDA National Nutrient Database, online at www.nal.usda.gov/fnic/foodcomp/search

2. Michelle Honda, Omega 3 Fatty Acids (EFAs) are Essential for Rebuilding Tissue and Improving Longevity. "Reverse Gut Diseases Naturally" 147-151; Retrieved Jan. 28, 2016.

3. Michelle Honda, Monitoring Candida Benefits All Gut Disorders. "Reverse Gut Diseases Naturally" 141-143; Retrieved Feb. 23, 2016.

Chapter 4

1. Alan R. Gaby, M.D. Nutritional Medicine. Fritz Perlberg Publishing; Concord, NH 2011. http://www.doctorgaby.com

2. Web MD. Vitamins that fight Inflammation. http://bit.ly/SK2H5C

4. C. Bhaskarsmand; G. Sadasivan. Effects of Feeding Irradiated Wheat to Malnourished Children. Am J Clin Nutr. 1975, 28:2, 130-5. http://ajcn.nutrition.org

5. S. E. Swithers. Artificial sweeteners produce a counterintuitive effect of inducing metabolic derangements. Trends in Endocrinology & Metabolism Journal. July 10, 2013. www.ncbi.nlm.nih.gov/

Chapter 5

1. Glycemic Index Testing. The University of Sydney. 2014. http://www.glycemicindex.com/testing_research.phpGlycemic Index Testing & Research

2. American Diabetes Association. http://www.diabetes.org/food-and-fitness/food/what-can-i-eat/understanding-carbohydrates/glycemic-index-and-diabetes.html?referrer=https://www.google.ca/

3. Mehta K, et al. Comparison of glucosamine sulfate and a polyherbal supplement (Maca Root) for the relief of osteoarthritis of the knee: a randomized controlled trial {ISRCTN25438351}. BMC Complement Altern Med. (2007)

4. Manikandan P, et al. Ocimum sanctum Linn. (Holy Basil - Tulsi) ethanolic leaf extract protects against 7, 12-dimethylbenz(a)anthrace ne-induced genotoxicity, oxidative stress, and imbalance in xenobiotic-metabolizing enzymes. J Med Food 2007; 10(3):495-502.

5. Bhattacharya S, et al. Hepatoprotective properties of kombucha tea against TBHP-induced oxidative stress via suppression of mitochondria dependent apoptosis. Pathophysiology 2011; 18:221–234.

Chapter 6

1. Top 12 Reasons To Take Omega 3 Fatty Acids. 2015,04:14. http://michelle-honda-blog.renewyou.ca/top-12-reasons-take-omega-3-fatty-acids-efas/

2. Best 5 Steps to Empower the Body to Heal. 2015,03:19. http://michelle-honda-blog.renewyou.ca/best-5-steps-empower-body-to-heal/

3. Zinc Second Most Important Mineral in the Body. 2015,05:20. http://michelle-honda-blog.renewyou.ca/zinc-second-most-important-mineral-body/

4. Magnesium - Vital for Crohn's Colitis IBS Mood Disorders. 2015,03:24 http://michelle-honda-blog.renewyou.ca/magnesium-vital-crohns-colitis-ibs-mood-disorders/

5. Iodine - Best Supplements for Health. 2015,09:23. http://michelle-honda-blog.renewyou.ca/iodine-best-supplements-for-health/

6. L-Tyrosine and Iodine - Main Energy Components. 2015,09:16. http://michelle-honda-blog.renewyou.ca/l-tyrosine-iodine-main-energy-components/

Chapter 7

1. Prior R, Wu X, Schaich K (2005) Standardized methods for the determination of antioxidant capacity and phenolics in foods and dietary supplements. J Argic Food Chem 53 (10):4290-4302. PMID 15884874

2. Blumberg JB, Frei B. Why clinical trials of vitamin E and cardiovascular diseases may be fatally flawed. Commentary on "The relationship between dose of vitamin E and suppression of oxidative stress in humans." Free Radic Biol Med 2007;43:1374-6. (PubMed abstract) https://ods.od.nih.gov/factsheets/VitaminE-HealthProfessional/

3. Cho SH, et al. Clinical efficacy and safety of Lyprinol, a patented extract from New Zealand green-lipped mussel (Perna canaliculus) in patients with osteoarthritis of the hip and knee: a multicenter 2-month clinical trial. European Annals of Allergy and Clinical Immunology. 2003;35:212-216.

4. Schauss AG et al. Journal of Agricultural and Food Chemistry, 2006A, 2006B

5. Laboratory analysis of hydrophilic ORAC value only (Brunswick Labs, 2005), Schauss, AG et al. Federation of Societies Experimental Biology Journal (2006)

Chapter 8

1. P. W. Tebbey, T. M. Buttke. Immunology, 1990 July; 70(3): 379–386

2. World Health Organization Quality of Medicines for Everyone, Contaminated magnesium stearate VG EP excipient manufactured by Ferro. Dec.22, 2011.

Chapter 9

1. Sasaki H, Sunagawa Y, Takahashi K, et al. Innovative preparation of Curcumin for improved oral bioavailability. Biol Pharm Bull. 2011;34(5):660-5.

2. Kimmatkar N, et al. Efficacy and tolerability of Boswellia serrata extract in treatment of osteoarthritis of knee a randomized double-blind placebo-controlled trial. Phytomedicine. 2003; 10:3-7.

3. Safayhi H, Rall B, Sailer ER, Ammon HP. Inhibition by boswellic acids of human leukocyte elastase. J Pharmacol Exp Ther. 1997 Apr;281(1):460-3.

4. Pilarski R, Zielinski H, Ciesiolka D, Gulewicz K. Antioxidant activity of ethanolic and aqueous extracts of Uncaria tomentosa (Cat's Claw); (Willd.) DC. J Ethnopharmacol. 2006 Mar 8;104(1-2):18-23.

5. Miller MJ, Ahmed S, Bobrowski P, Haqqi TM. The chrondoprotective actions of a natural product are associated with the activation of IGF-1 production by human chondrocytes despite the presence of IL-1beta. BMC Complement Altern Med. 2006 Apr 7;6:13.

6. Lenfeld J Motl O Trka A. Anti-inflammatory activity of extracts from Conyza Canadensis. PHARMAZIE 1986 Apr; 41(4):268-9.

7. Eichler et al: Antiphlogistic, analgesic and spasmolytic effect of harpagoside, a glycoside from the root of Harpagophytum procumbens. ARZNEIUM FORSCH (Jan 70) 20 (1): 107-9.

8. Shimizu et al. Combination effects of Shosaikoto (Chinese traditional medicine) and prednisolone on the anti-inflammatory action. J PHARMACOBIODYN 1984 Dec; 7(12):891-9.

9. Sinomenium acutum: Eur Rev Med Pharmacol Sci. 2012 Sep;16(9):1184-91. Anti-inflammatory effect of sinomenine by inhibition of pro-inflammatory mediators in PMA plus A23187-stimulated HMC-1 Cells.

10. Aihua Zhang, Hui Sun, Xijun Wang. Recent advances in natural products from plants for treatment of liver. European Journal of Medicinal Chemistry: 63(2013) 570-577.

11. Anti-Inflammatory and Antinociceptive Activities of Anthraquinone-2-Carboxylic Acid. Jae Gwang Park,1 Seung Cheol Kim; Volume 2016 (2016), Article ID 1903849, 12 pages. http://dx.doi.org/10.1155/2016/1903849

12. Skullcap, Kudo: Studies on Scutellariae radix.V11. Anti-arthritic and anti-inflammatory actions of methanolic extract and flavoniod components from Scutellariae radix. CHEM PHARM BULL (TOKYO) (1984 Jul) 32(7):2724-9

Chapter 10

1. Jensen, Bernard. Foods That Heal. Avery Publishing Group Inc. 1993.

2. Roger C. Rinn, PhD. Ralph E. Carson PhD. Harnessing the Healing Power of Fruit. 2008.

ABOUT THE AUTHOR

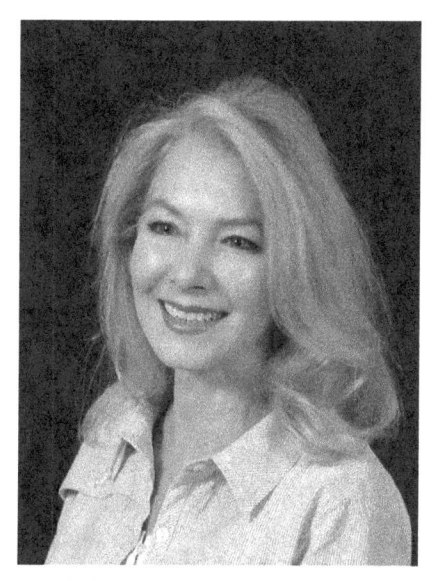

Michelle Honda, Ph.D. is a holistic doctor who specializes in disease reversal through the employment of natural medicine and clinical nutrition. Within two years of finishing her Ph.D., Michelle opened a Holistic Health Clinic with her husband Ron Honda, called Renew You Holistic Health (www.renewyou.ca) in Ancaster, Ontario, Canada, where she conducts her private practice.

The author of the innovative book *Reverse Gut Disease Naturally*, Michelle is an author who is wholly devoted to the welfare of mankind and the preservation of the environment. Her success in full disease reversal of intestinal complaints is unprecedented, and she has developed a reputation for being an expert in the field of applied natural medicine and clinical nutrition.

Michelle has applied this same expertise to *Reverse Heart Disease Naturally*, as well as the latest series addition *Reverse Inflammation Naturally*. Michelle is passionate about sharing the sort of knowledge that offers readers the power of personal choice, enabling others to restore, renew and rejuvenate themselves. To this end, Michelle continues to publish informative articles enlightening others on their journey to wellness.

Visit her website at www.michellehonda.com.

Also in the *Hatherleigh Natural Health Guides* Series

Reverse Gut Diseases Naturally
ISBN 978-1-57826-596-1

Reverse Heart Disease Naturally
ISBN 978-157826-663-0

Available at www.hatherleighpress.com and wherever books are sold.